a MEMoiR OF LoVE AND MADNESS

Living with bipolar disorder

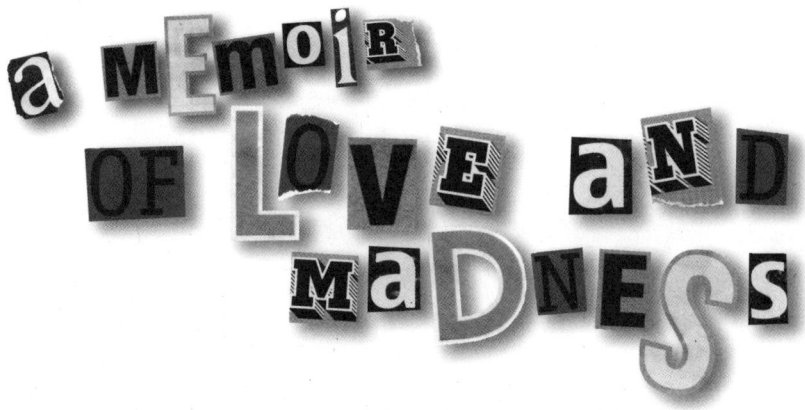

a memoir of love and madness

Living with bipolar disorder

Rahla Xenopoulos

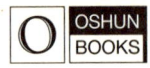

Published by Oshun Books
an imprint of Random House Struik (Pty) Ltd
Company Reg. No. 1966/003153/07
80 McKenzie Street, Cape Town, 8001
PO Box 1144, Cape Town, 8000, South Africa

www.oshunbooks.co.za

First published 2009

1 3 5 7 9 10 8 6 4 2

Publication © Oshun Books 2009
Text © Rahla Xenopoulos 2009

Cover photograph: Jonathan Harris/Back cover photograph: Fiona McPherson

PUBLISHER: Marlene Fryer
MANAGING EDITOR: Ronel Richter-Herbert
EDITOR: Roxanne Reid
PROOFREADER: Ronel Richter-Herbert
COVER AND TEXT DESIGNER: Monique Oberholzer
TYPESETTER: Monique van den Berg
PRODUCTION MANAGER: Valerie Kömmer

Set in 12 pt on 16 pt Bembo

Reproduction by Hirt & Carter (Cape) (Pty) Ltd
Printed and bound by Pinetown Printers, Pinetown, KwaZulu-Natal

ISBN 978 1 77020 025 8

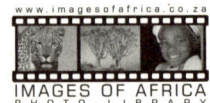

To Jason ... my beginning, my middle, my everlasting

Contents

Acknowledgements

pninadavidgigijonty-lviahgerald,
the Fenster family for their divine inspiration and humour

The triplets, Gidon Greg, Layla Tallulah and Samuel Jacob,
my daily reminder that there is a God and that miracles do occur

Anne,
the angel of my every word

Shauna, Mary, Ronel and Roxanne,
my shepherds

Dr Leigh Janet,
for introducing me to life in this world

Foreword

Rahla has a very serious disorder – I know from personal experience, when she set fire to my closest friend. It is a miracle she was able to lift a pen rather than swallow it. So, just for being able to sit up for so long, I think she deserves to sell if not one, then at least three of her books. Please, I beg you to help her – she might be a genius. Considering she's nuts, she can write like a dream.

As someone who comes from the dark side mentally, she makes me feel not so alone.

Ruby Wax

Prelude

It's 4 a.m. and my brain is buzzing, ideas swarming and galloping through my head, bombarding me with their imagined brilliance. I've been up all night, writing poetry and dancing to the Waterboys' 'The Whole of the Moon'. I've tried phoning everyone I know, but everyone I know is asleep. All around me is silence – even the birds are silent – an overwhelming stillness that provides a startling counterpoint to the hullabaloo going on inside my brain. There's no one out there, no one can touch me, I fly too high, I wear a shield of mania.

Just a few days later and I crash into darkness, a resounding fall. Thud. No poems, no ideas, no energetic dances. Nothing inside me but the ache of sadness, stagnant, silent, reverberating from my stomach throughout my body. Each sound, the tip-tap of the dogs' paws on wooden floors, the phone's incessant ringing, the whoosh of passing cars, every sound is an assault, a shrill shriek puncturing my fractured nerves, flaying them raw. I'm shut away in a place too dark, too narrow for anyone else to enter. I crouch behind a macabre wall of pain that no one can penetrate. I am empty, desolate and utterly alone.

I can't say that bipolar disorder has made my life easy, but it has educated me, and it has certainly humbled me. It's made me vulnerable and forced me to tell the truth at times when lies would have tripped more willingly from my lips.

But sickness is our cure. On days when I've thought, 'So this is it, surely now I can't take another breath,' I've discovered that illness comes with inner resources and a strength that none of us knows we have until life forces us to find them. It has cured me of inertia and it has compelled me to live a healthy, disciplined life. It has thrown me into violent chaos and forced me to be a serious person, when I wanted to be a homecoming queen.

Some days, regardless of the weather, it has compelled me to see gloomy grey clouds outside my window … and on other days, it has had me, a mad person, flying about, chasing summers long since past. So, while sickness certainly has not been a pleasant companion these past forty years, it has somehow been poetic.

This book is about a girl who grew up in a warm and eccentric family of brilliant people always committed to helping her. Even when no one knew what was actually wrong with her, they carried her through anorexia, bulimia, episodes of unmanageable mania and financial ruin. They held her close through deep depression, three suicide attempts and years of self-mutilation.

It is also the story of a girl who fell in love with a tall, dark stranger from a faraway land, a stranger whose arms became her home – a home in which she danced, sang out loud (with an abominable voice), cried even louder, laughed, and struggled for years to have a child.

This is the story of a girl who was on Ritalin from the age of seven, who had dyslexia and remedial problems and was hyperactive. After failing two years, she dropped out of high school to become a career psychiatric patient. But then, of course, love arrived, as did a doctor with the correct diagnosis, a combination of drugs that worked … and, finally, the call of blank pages that wanted words on them.

In the story that follows there's no rigidly chronological structure. It is a collection of the themes of my life, because this is how my mind works, how I remember things. Now I fear the time has come for me to read what's already been written, and I'm afraid I'll be put off writing because of the awkwardness of the sentence structure, the clunky vocabulary and the frivolous self-centredness. My trembling hand will never again find the page. It's such a tenuous thread, the yarn that keeps me writing, as tenuous as my link to sanity. But then the sun comes out, the camellias blossom and the empty page beckons.

Don't be fooled into thinking that this story about madness is a sad one. No – it's about love and happy endings! I wasn't a writer when I set out to write this book; I was just a girl, at times too sad to brush my teeth, at times too insane to eat. At times I was amused, but always I was in love and, most of the time, I was grateful.

Popular psychology teaches us to aspire to a state of balance. How to do this has always confounded me, because there's no balance in the known world. Not in its seasons or geography, or even in our very bodies with their strange biorhythms and propensity for growth. Life doesn't meander along on a well-balanced, staid path.

For the best and the boldest of us, it's a hell of an unpredictable ride.

This is in no way an apology for the structure, or lack thereof, in my life, but the truth is, as much as I'd like to have written a neat, concise story, with a beginning, a middle and an end, well, my life just hasn't afforded me one. Instead, my life continues on its insanely, predictably unpredictable path. Dreams fail me, and dreams come true.

CHAPTER 1

The Happy Potter doctor

For some reason, mania comes to me around November – well, September to November. I think my first full-blown manic episode happened just before my twentieth birthday. I had gone on a teenage crash diet, which I found surprisingly easy to maintain. For days I got by on precious little food or sleep. But I baked constantly. While listening to 'alternative' songs on Radio Metro at 4 a.m. I mixed and muddled chocolate brownies I had no intention of eating.

I was always the life and soul of the party. I didn't sleep around, but I was the most flirtatious, irrepressible, confident and boundlessly energetic girl standing or dancing, usually surrounded by a sea of men. I'd wake up laughing. It was as if I had X-ray vision into people's souls. I could see through the layers of their facades, their protective devices, their pain and dreams. It was extraordinary.

I taught life skills and drama to street children at a home in Hillbrow. After teaching, I'd walk through 'The Brow' at night, past its trendy shopfronts. I never felt threatened by the desperate outcasts who lived there – street urchins and homeless schizophrenics. I'd stop and look down the ominous dark alleys, seeking out stoned victims, drunk criminals and corrupt policemen who seemed to whisper and whimper in a chorus. Fearless, I was 'Little Miss S in her mini dress/Living it up to die'. In a short skirt and Doc Martens I'd stomp down to a crummy building, up a dirty staircase and into a flat, where I was greeted by the misery of a poster depicting a beaten woman, who had at her feet the words, 'Sister, we bleed ...'

Among the trampled and the battered, the feminists and the healers, I counselled at POWA (People Opposing Women Abuse). At the time, it seemed to me that when I wasn't partying, this was a pretty normal way to spend an evening. I was tireless and unstoppable. I thought I was immortal. Boy, did I have delusions of grandeur.

Invariably, with this level of overexcitement, with this mania, came the dancing, which has always had a way of pushing me over the edge. I can never just dance as a casual hobby. It has to be an intense experience. Reflected in a studio mirror, floor to ceiling, wall to wall, I expect to see the grace of the human form lifted effortlessly in rhythmic free flight.

The sad irony is that I am not a born, or a natural, dancer. No matter how much I starve myself, my body will always be the wrong shape. Short of limb, lumpy of frame, I've found myself at times to be either too big of breast or too wide of girth. My brain is dyslexic, so I find myself confused, slow, and at times even dancing in the wrong direction. But I'm passionate, and passion can propel a girl into many a pirouette nature never intended her to achieve. After gruelling hours of practice I was sometimes rewarded with a fleeting moment of magnificence, when the music inhabited my clumsy human form and my body drifted and glided gloriously through the primal freedom of dance.

During that first November mania, as my body weight just about halved and my personality changed, it never occurred to me that something might be wrong. Everything felt profoundly *right*. I didn't feel detached or unreal; I felt more myself than ever. It was as if, for my whole life, I'd been allowed only privileged glimpses of the real Rahla, and suddenly that was who I was *all the time*. I had no reason to believe the feeling would pass. It was fabulous, and I was hysterical and ecstatic with me-ness. And I kept getting thinner and thinner.

What happened next is a bit of a blur. Let's see. I did a neuro-linguistic programming workshop, which ended with a fire-walk. Perhaps that is what pushed me over the edge into a state of pure, divine mania. On the other hand, I did another fire-walk a few years later and didn't get remotely manic. When it's gonna come, it's gonna come, and that's that.

Time passed. After the long night of baking, I flew high and got dumped low. I went to insane places, but I never lived in *this* world. A few doctors tried to help. When I was manic, I wouldn't eat or sleep, and so, at the age of twenty-three, a doctor diagnosed me with anorexia. Two years later, reluctantly crawling through the aftermath of mania and falling into its ensuing depression, I found myself hankering after the hollow high of mania. The next doctor diagnosed bulimia. Even with the best intentions in the world, no one could establish what was wrong with me.

Then, at the ripe old age of twenty-eight, after the fun and games of another manic episode, I finally agreed to see a highly thought-of doctor to get a professional opinion on my state of mind. I felt there was nothing he could tell me that I didn't already know. Here I was,

I told myself, serenely enlightened and conscientisised. All my life I'd been prodded and studied, analysed and paralysed. I'd been a hyperactive child, dyslexic, remedial, anorexic, bulimic. I'd been a rebel and a late bloomer. I'd had attention deficit disorder and I'd had depression. What was this doctor going to tell me that could possibly add to that list?

I sat in his waiting room and watched children play while their dysfunctional mothers consulted the great doctor. I flipped casually through outdated magazines. I was way cool, so much cleverer than all this. I'd already told my darkest secrets to dotty dopeheads in candlelit rooms. I'd done Eastern healing, Western healing; I'd stood on my head and leapt off my toes.

But the truth was that nothing had really helped. I knew something else was wrong with me, something that did not seem to have a name. Secretly, I dreaded the idea of telling this strange doctor my diary of disorders. I was funny and irreverent about it, but it was still painful. And for all the witty labels I gave myself, it was also embarrassing.

I picked up another magazine. Boring. Then I read a paragraph of the book I took from my handbag, but couldn't concentrate, so I put it back. I went to the bathroom and reapplied my lipstick, slowly, with a miniature gold brush and lipliner. Still no sign of the famous doctor; where was the man? Again I opened my bag, taking out my miniature diary and gazing at the empty little pages, pretending to write down appointments with my miniature pen.

Waiting, agitating, I started to get annoyed; I had to go home and rearrange the flowers, make dinner. Who did he think he was to keep me waiting so long? I thought about leaving, simply walking out and going home. Then he came smiling down the corridor, looking like a cheerful Teletubby. He guided me to his disordered office, filled with opened books, closed books and photographs that faced away from me. He sat down. On his crowded desk was a prescription pad and jars of pens and pencils, and paperweights advertising drug companies. I nervously leant over, picking up a Montblanc pen. It didn't work. As if from far away, I heard his words. They fell out of his mouth with random matter-of-factness. 'You're bipolar and you have obsessive–compulsive tendencies. But you know that, of course.'

I baulked. Obviously the man was mad. Who did he think he was, flippantly announcing such a dramatic diagnosis? I wanted a CAT scan. I wanted proof, pictures. For the love of God, I'm a product of the age of proof, not the age of instinct!

'What is "bipolar" anyway?' I wondered, not sure I wanted to know. 'Does that mean I'm a polar Eskimo who sleeps with both men and women?' Facetious. Was he telling me I was insane? Did he think I'd murder my family in their sleep? Did he want to have me institutionalised? I pictured myself as Frances Farmer; could I insist on a Gucci straightjacket? Did Gucci make a straightjacket?

Images of Jeff Levy flashed before me, the local lunatic of my childhood who had always been in love with my sister Gigi and who, after burning down his family home and being placed in an asylum, woke up every Sunday at 5 a.m. to make the hour-and-a-half trek, barefoot and insane, all the way to our family home to see her. He'd been diagnosed schizophrenic.

I'd never met anyone who was bipolar (what they used to call manic depressive) or who had obsessive–compulsive disorder or obsessive–compulsive personality disorder. At least, not that I knew of. None of my boyfriends had casually slipped the words, 'PS. I'm certifiably insane,' into my mouth with the first kiss.

This was silly. Sure, I'm somewhat hither and thither; some days I wake up inside out and go to sleep upside down, but heavens, surely he wasn't saying I was barking mad?

I swallowed back the vomit suddenly in my mouth. Consternation. All of the pens suddenly leapt from their jars. Some were in my mouth, in my hands, behind my ear, drawing on a notepad in front of me. Oh, for goodness sake, I wasn't mad. I just had curly hair.

I looked up and noticed that this doctor had kind, perhaps even intelligent, eyes. He started explaining things, asking pertinent questions and offering behavioural descriptions. I started wondering about my 'eccentric' obsession with miniaturising my world. Very much against my will, I began to recognise aspects of what he was saying. Maybe there was some truth in this new diagnosis.

I'd always had what I thought of as my little 'idiosyncracies'. People used to laugh at my cupboards, for instance. Rows upon rows of white and gold Chanel boxes (bought during manic shopping binges) categorised into little families. Hosiery, for example. Box one: dancing. Box two: laddered. Box three: black, thick. Box four: pantyhose. Box five: stockings and suspenders. Box six: coloured. 'Boxing', so to speak, gave me a sense of order. All my clothing, down to my underwear, was colour-coordinated.

I also had a thing about physical symmetry. Sensations had to be duplicated on both sides of my body, so if someone squeezed my right hand, I had to have my left hand squeezed in precisely the same way. Dancing could drive me mad – step-ball-change and spin to the right; I'd have to pinch my left leg to stop it from leaping step-ball-change and spin to the left.

And there was more. My universe had to be miniaturised. All meals were served out of a christening set. I ate breakfast from a little teething cup with two quaint handles, dinner on a little-bitty plate. My tiny clutch bag contained a small Filofax in which I wrote microscopic words with a baby pen. I'd thought this penchant for small things, neatness and symmetry was cute, slightly odd, nothing more. The doctor thought otherwise.

Cringing, reluctantly, I recalled the malicious laughing voice I'd never told anyone about, that of an imagined phantasm, an old man, whose presence had terrified me since childhood. 'Ha, ha, ha.' Maybe the term bipolar explained certain things, like those times of invincible euphoria that would later crumble into a despair so deep that no one could reach me. I was trying to force myself to listen to the doctor. I wanted to know more; I didn't want to know another thing.

He was saying that there was something really wrong with me, but he hadn't carried out any tests, so how could he be sure? No! I couldn't stay, I wouldn't listen, and I wouldn't accept any of it. I was out of there.

In an enraged fury I drove to my parents' house. I drove badly. The sound of cars hooting followed me all the way home. My parents were in the study, reading. I stormed in, complaining, crying with rage. 'I hate the doctor. He's a buffoon! He didn't even talk to me, didn't treat me as a whole person. Just threw a diagnosis at me. He probably calls all of his patients bipolar! It must be a trendy new illness.'

I was beside myself with rage and in total denial. I insisted that my father complain on my behalf. The doctor was too modern, too chemical, not holistic, really not a legitimate psychiatrist at all; in fact, more of a carpenter. He treated me like a block of wood to be chopped up or carved into pieces; he should be struck off the medical roll. My voice rose in indignation.

This wasn't the way I wanted my life to go. I was in love and I wanted my boyfriend Jason to marry me. I wanted to have babies and live happily ever after. How could I lead any kind of meaningful or enjoyable life if I took on this exotic diagnosis? It was a witch-hunt, a conspiracy. Sure, I'd done some pretty dippy things in my life, but I was an ordinary girl, ordinary girl, ordinary girl.

My mother and father appeared calm. Everything stayed in its place. Rows and rows of books wallpapered the room. The side tables were stained with the rings of coffee cups, as they had been since my childhood. I escaped into the comfort of our domestic worker Melita's room. She was knitting, as she always had since I was small. I climbed up onto her bed, which was raised with bricks to keep away the *tokoloshe*. The room smelt of wool, of the jerseys Melita had made for me all my life – wool and Nivea cream, little blue jars of Nivea cream that she used lovingly to apply to my face when I was a child.

In the enveloping familiarity and comfort of her smell, I finally took a deep breath and quietly admitted to myself that maybe the doctor was right. I was bipolar and, undoubtedly, I had obsessive–compulsive tendencies. I was with the right doctor, the Happy Potter doctor – thus named for his magic abilities, his mysterious insight and his wand of psychotropic miracles.

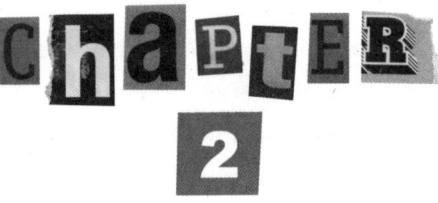

CHAPTER 2

The old man

Going right back into a time of innocence and helplessness, I have a bleak memory. I remember being curled up in a foetal position under an overstuffed Victorian armchair, tugging nervously at the strands of yarn I'd managed to pry loose from the upholstery above my head. I remember the agony of discovering that even in a confined space, my improvised fort, I couldn't hide from the sneering old man, just as I couldn't hide from the enormous sadness that sometimes invaded my small frame. I remember my mother crouching down to hug me. I remember feeling inconsolable. I remember the old man not going away.

The old man. This isn't a person I'd talk about in therapy, not something I'd divulge to my best friend over cappuccinos or mention on a date. The old man is weird, awful; a voice, a vision, one of the most violent features of my life. He appears when all hope is lost and all that's wholesome and good has deserted me. When I'm shredded and bewildered, the old man is there to taunt me.

I suppose I was about five years old when I first became aware of him. In front of the dining room was a patio with a makeshift 'roof' of wooden lattice. That day, the sun shone and the trellis was over-hung with wisteria, wafting lilac colours and fragrance over my curly head. I don't remember having any toys in front of me; I was playing with Tania, my ever-present imaginary friend.

At the time my family had an unkempt dog named Bundle, who rather resembled a bear. He would leap up onto the lattice above the patio and sprawl there while we ate alfresco below. Bundle could cause an uproar at a Sunday luncheon. But that morning it wasn't Bundle who interrupted my childish games.

I suddenly felt something hovering over me, and an eerie chill went through me. Life went into spooky slow motion; my every move, placing a hand in front of my face to look at the fingers, checking, slowly, slowly, yes, each one, all five, all there. I sensed something or someone looking down on me, slurring through my consciousness. I became quite still, too afraid to look up. Then I heard the distinct sound of laughter. Ugly laughter. No one there to protect me; even my imaginary friend Tania had vanished. Funny thing that: we don't control our imaginary friends – or our imagin-ary enemies.

Fearfully, reluctantly, I looked up at the wisteria blossoms and saw the gnarled, gaunt face of an old man laughing at me. It was a loud, theatrical laugh, 'Ha, Ha, Ha!' Although the laughter came from above my little head, it seemed to inhabit my entire body, witnessing my shame.

Shame about what? The laughter mocked my silly, childish games, my imaginary friend, my lack of real friends, my inability to stop sucking my thumb, my fear of Spike Milligan's Badjelly the Witch. My fear of sleeping in a room without my siblings, my fear of the dark, my petty fibs and peculiarities, even the way my little heart was pumping so fast when the world around me seemed to be moving so slowly.

The old man's laughter brought shame to the way I liked to wear my Laura Ashley party dress to painting classes, hem too long, trailing behind me in the dirt. Shame that my friend Brian and I had hidden behind the bunk bed and eaten my sister's Smarties. Why should a small child feel shame? I was engulfed by it, too helpless to defend myself, to say, 'I'm just an ordinary little girl and you're nothing, just a figment of my imagination. Poof, go away, go to pot.'

It's all fine and well to describe this now, but some days, well, I'm still too small and vulnerable to face the old man, and maybe it's just the saddest thing in my world.

It would be comforting to think that aliens had abducted me as some sort of absurd explanation for the apparition. But of course that's not the case. Instead, I'm periodically visited by – or, in psychological terms, I conjure up – an awful vision: the sound of an old man who laughs at me. I imagine a Jungian analyst would have a field day with me and my archetype of an old man whose awful laughter penetrates into the very marrow of my brittle bones. He arrives, not with a Tarantino-like violence or a Tom Waits lyrical and ironic sadness; no, he comes swirling out of nowhere with a contempt and a rage that is so ugly and other, so apart from me as I know myself. He haunts another girl in me, a girl who is damaged, weathered and worn out. He turns up very occasionally, and only when things are at their very bleakest – when there's not a ray of light in the sky.

Fortunately, he comes alone (although I imagine his partner Suicide is tagging behind somewhere), and he doesn't give me any instructions on how to live my life, no barked orders or mysterious commands. He's never filled me with religious zeal. He's just frightened and diminished me, causing me to forget who I am, to lose my bearings and my grip, not just on reality and self-worth, but also on my life force.

When I'm 'up', I resound as high and magnificent as a towering wave, but inevitably I crash – and the old man's always lurking nearby to laugh at the ensuing chaos. I can go for years without hearing from him, until I begin to hope he's gone, gone to the North Pole, where it snows and they have Christmas, gone where the goblins go, hey ho, hey ho. Then he reappears when my self-esteem is shrivelled up, when I'm a very small person curled up inside a thimble, so small and vulnerable that I scarcely exist. My skin thin, my nerves raw. When every car on the freeway seems aimed like a weapon poised to crash into me, when the falling of the Twin Towers can go unnoticed, the blooming of camellias unobserved.

When I've departed for a place where nothing and nobody can reach me, then, somehow, he finds me, curled up, hiding on the floor in the tiny nook underneath my dressing table with a chair to hide my fractured form. Rocking to and fro, to and fro, hither and thither, all helter-skelter, nothing is orderly; I am dislocated, disordered, falling apart – and I hear him roaring, 'Ha, Ha, Ha!'

My inner world speeds up and the outer world slows down. Like Jimi Hendrix screeching on a painful cocaine guitar, there's no melody, no symphony, no quiet refrain. Only that unbearable laughter, jeering at me, making me cringe. I have no idea what his appearance means or what he wants from me.

I don't know how he gets inside me. Like Dracula zooming in with exposed fangs through taboos of raw garlic, brandished crucifixes and a circle of my own personal protective Holy Crusaders, my laughing old man invades uninvited. He can penetrate medication and Chinese tinctures. *Nothing* keeps him away. He belittles and diminishes me, and I have never lashed out at the intrusion, never confronted him and challenged, 'You have no place here! What do you want from me?'

My old man seems satisfied just to be there, laughing mirthlessly, thinking, 'Rahla Marilyn Fenster, you are a failure, you are nothing, a nobody, a waste of society's resources! You've never achieved anything and you never will. You've never held down a job, earned any money you could hold on to. Every time you begin doing something worthwhile, you manifest a crying germ.'

A crying germ is like flu. Except instead of sneezing and being snotty, I just cry. Flu doesn't respond to quick fixes; it responds to days in bed, hot toddies and chicken soup. So, too, with crying germs. I have to wait out the depression. I cry at people, strangers mostly, because it seems as if they all hate me: the people at the bank, the ladies working in the shop, everyone in the world. The safest thing is to take to my bed and cry, 'Waah, waah, waah.' And then, like flu, it slowly drifts out of my system until, finally, my body is all cried out. It's a germ, a crying germ.

The old man would continue to mock me. 'What is actually wrong with you anyway? If you're so sick, where's the blood? Where are the X-rays showing broken bones or fluid on the lungs? Face it, you're fabricating the whole thing to get attention. You're not a fully functioning member of this universe. You might as well be dead. Everyone is watching you and it's all really *very* funny – Ha, Ha, Ha!'

Sure, this is me talking, it's me projecting. The old man doesn't exist, not really. The laughter is my own self-taunting invention. But when that harsh resounding laughter crashes down on me, erupts from above and within, then I become nothing. The summer garden around me doesn't help, the sound of the sea or the birds singing fades away. I can't string beads, talk, write or take enough drugs to drive him away. He hovers there, floating above and around me, laughing, gloating.

Even though I now know that this vile old man is a product of my own deranged mind, a part of me goes on believing that perhaps he's my punishment. Maybe he's there to remind me that, in the end, I'll always be nothing more than a broken girl.

When I'm good, I'm grand, and when I'm not, I manage just, only just, to survive. And I'm grateful just to survive. Forget Joan of Arc. There's no bright side to hearing voices and seeing visions. There are a lot of jokes about it – it's a subject susceptible to good jokes and, God knows, I'm always up for one. But I'd rather not talk about this than make light of it, because it's so terrifying, so dark, so *not* funny. I can't put on a brave face, because the reality for me is appalling.

It's the ultimate cruelty and the ultimate sensation of losing all control precisely because it's a torture that comes from within; my mind turning on itself. That my mind was capable of victimising me in this way when I was just a child makes me so very sad for that little girl playing under the wisteria.

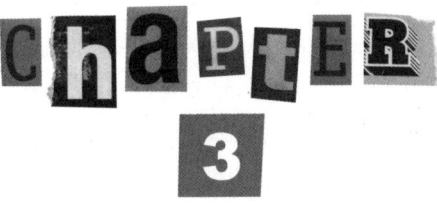

CHAPTER 3

Family Fenster

When it comes to family memories, my inner eye – the one that takes pictures of what happened and then stores them for future reference – goes into soft focus. Everything becomes pink and hazy with the sound of children laughing, as if captured within the jumping, jagged movements of a home movie, lovingly spliced together.

Like a looking glass, the inner eye recalls children skipping through the rainbows formed by sprinklers gushing water onto lawns. Maybe my happiest inaccuracies lie predominantly among my family, even though we were and remain picture-book perfect. Happier and better adjusted and more in love with one another than all the sitcoms we grew up watching: *The Brady Bunch*, *Eight Is Enough*, even *The Cosby Show*.

Pnina is my pretty oldest sister. In childhood, I used to stare at her long chestnut hair while she lay sleeping, like a princess from a faraway land. I could stare at her undisturbed for hours, because we five children all slept in the same bedroom. It probably wasn't for long that we shared, but it was so fabulous that the memory dominates my childhood recollections.

Mr Makepiece, the carpenter, had put together a wonderful assemblage of beds built within beds and cupboards hidden behind drawers, a spiralled maze of delight in which we explored, played and slept. This magical bed–cupboard system meant my sister Gigi's head was positioned at my feet, and she used to make up stories with my toes. Each toe was given a name and had a character. Pnina told us stories about the nightly adventures of a funny little fellow named Sanna. He was the shadow cast by a torch after the lights had been turned out, and his adventures were predominantly mischievous.

Mr Makepiece was a grateful patient who paid my father with household construction and repairs for his psychiatric services. My father often worked on a kind of barter system so that, while cash didn't abound, at times we'd have a surplus of crocheted blankets, chocolate cakes, even watches. All manner of people needed psychiatric care, and some of them couldn't afford it.

Another patient of the barter system was Fernando, who had the biggest hands I'd ever seen. He could hold the world in them.

Every Pesach, the holiday when we Jews celebrate our release as slaves from Egypt with a rather sombre menu (lest, God forbid, we should forget our bitter tears), we eat unleavened bread. Every year of my childhood, at Pesach, Fernando arrived at the front door carrying cardboard boxes filled with groceries. Excited, we children would empty the boxes onto the dining-room table and find chocolates, bottles of sweet wine and matzos, all of it kosher for Passover.

Months later, on Rosh Hashanah, the holiday when we celebrate the coming of the New Year, the menu is a festive affair of round bread filled with raisins, and apples dipped in honey to symbolise the sweetness and roundness we anticipate for the New Year. (Religious symbolism is explained in the food, indicating the great priority food has in our lives.)

Fernando would again arrive, carrying large cardboard boxes filled with groceries in his Herculean hands. Delighted, we children would dig in and, again, out would spill chocolates, bottles of sweet wine and matzos, all of it kosher. It was a great mystery to us all – how did Fernando find Passover food six months after Passover?

In the Tuscan region of Campania there's a medieval town called Pietrelcina. Living in the friary of San Giovanni Rotondo was a modest yet great monk. His name was Padre Pio, and he bore the stigmata. People came from all over Italy to seek solace and spiritual guidance from this humble man, who exuded serenity and endured the pains of his wounds and spontaneous bleeding with great courage. He inspired faith and tranquillity in his many followers.

Fernando's parents were simple, good people. When their son was consumed by a strange illness, a dark madness they couldn't understand, they went to see the Padre. He told Fernando's parents that the family would journey to a land far away with a hot climate, where they would find a healer with a small, pretty wife who would have long black hair and look Italian. This healer would cure their son.

It was the 1950s, and my father had just qualified as a psychiatrist. He was doing his internship at Tara, the state-owned psychiatric hospital in Johannesburg. One Monday morning he was greeted by what must have appeared to be extras from a Fellini film. Sitting still and stiff-backed was a painfully thin man in a carefully darned evening suit; on his lap he clutched a faded black hat. A stout woman fidgeted nervously with a rosary. Between them slouched a large teenager, who seemed to have a shadow of sadness lurking over him. There was no problem with breaking the ice, or working through boundaries and trust issues, or any of the usual social awkwardness. Barely able to speak English, the couple greeted my father with a rehearsed barrage of questions:

Italian father: We would like to know, are you a married doctor?
Daddy: Yes, I am a married doctor.
Italian wife: *Bene, bene*, Doctor. This is a good sign.
Italian father: Your wife, she has pale hair or dark hair?
Daddy (taken aback but amused by the interest in his wife): My wife has long black hair.
Italian wife: *Bene, bene*, Doctor, this is good.
(The anxiety in the surgery was lifting considerably; this was developing into a very successful session.)
Italian father: Your dark wife, she is beautiful or ugly?
Daddy: She's renowned for her great beauty!
Italian wife: *Bene, bene*, Doctor, this is good.
Italian father: She is small or she is large?
Daddy: She is petite.
Italian wife: *Bene, bene*, Doctor, this is good.
Italian father: Please, you must invite us to eat at your home tonight.

Unethical as it may have been to invite the first patients on a Monday morning into his home that evening, my father typically went along with the odd request. They were strangers in a strange land, and the son's sad expression hadn't altered at all during the animated exchange.

And so it was that my beautiful, dark, petite mother with her long black hair caught up in a Mediterranean-looking braid, wearing a

Frida Kahlo skirt and carrying a baby on each hip, opened the front door to the Italian family. The wife took one look at her, fell to the ground and kissed the hem of my astonished mother's skirt. The father wept and said, 'You, Doctor, you will cure my son. We have come all the way to Africa for you to cure my son!'

The following morning Daddy returned to his office to make his tragic diagnosis. The boy Fernando was schizophrenic. Hardly a curable illness even today, but back in 1959 it was hopeless. Despite the predictions of the great Padre, my father couldn't cure the boy, and after a while he was transferred to Sterkfontein, an institution for the severely mentally ill. There he was left to languish, catatonic and barely conscious, hopeless among other incurables, for a few years, till my father happened to be posted to Sterkfontein.

A drug company wanting to perform controlled drug tests on the schizophrenic patients approached Daddy. Twenty patients were given the new drug, and twenty were given a placebo. Neither doctor nor patient was allowed to know who was given the placebo and who was given the drug.

At the end of the trial, out of the forty patients, only one re-sponded – Fernando. He emerged generous, expansive and light, constantly brimming with gratitude. Gratitude to my father, to the Padre, to Jesus, to the universe and to the miracle of each new day.

The funny thing was that, many years later, when all was said and done, when Padre Pio had been canonised and Fernando had had children and grandchildren of his own, the hospital records were disclosed and my father discovered that Fernando had been given the placebo.

To my childish eyes, Fernando exuded a magnificent glow. I think it was the glow of faith. Faith that there exist priests whose hands inexplicably bleed, faith that such a priest can miraculously predict an encounter in a faraway land with a doctor and his beautiful wife, faith that even the most godforsaken sicknesses can sometimes find cures.

All my life, Fernando seemed backlit. We'd open the front door to a man with a permanent smile on his face and the sun shining warm upon his back. The smell of grapes lingered around him as he hummed the romantic old tune 'Mamma', as sung by the tenor Beniamino Gigli. *Of course* Fernando could procure fresh matzos on Rosh Hashanah! Fields of sunflowers turned away from the sun to gaze at him. He could find that place somewhere over the rainbow where the bluebirds sing. He could do anything. People who have returned from the dark always can.

I adored both my funny, protective sisters, but my big brother David was my king. Why I couldn't marry him when I grew up was a mystery to me. When it was time for David's bar mitzvah, I made him a crown and mud cakes. He wore the crown for a little while before the party, but didn't eat the cakes. Later in life he became a hippie. He had a mane of curly brown hair like Samson's, and, like Samson, he refused to cut it short. He wore ripped jeans, played a lot of pinball and listened to rock music. He played the drums and the piano magnificently, and had inherited Daddy's wicked sense of humour. Girls loved him passionately.

Then David became religious. He continued to listen to rock music, wear ripped jeans, and play the drums and piano. Girls continued to love him. I think he may have cut down on the pinball, though. But he dropped out of university, where he was studying social work, and went to a yeshiva to study. He met Evida, a gentle, soft-spoken, wise girl who understood not only him, but his whole daft family. They were married when she was eighteen and he was twenty.

Years later someone told me that the first time he saw David swaying backwards and forwards in devout meditative prayer in Synagogue, he'd assumed he must have been stoned off his head. But that wasn't the case. David is that rare phenomenon, the real deal. He's still the gentlest, most humane person I've ever known, incapable of malice. At the yeshiva, he studied to become a rabbi. When he and his friends came to visit us, they used to bring their own food and eat off paper plates, because our food wasn't kosher. David constantly drummed, even with plastic utensils on the dining-room table.

My brother Jonty was a boy with a funny dance. He loved fast cars, but our family never had any. He was popular and funny. Jonty worked out at the gym and went to a lot of parties. Unlike me, he managed, with great exuberance, to crack the King David school social structure while remaining himself – a bit crazy and a lot funny.

If I needed help, a shoulder to cry on, a lift to a party or an account to be settled, he never failed to come through for me. But later he would consider my stoned, ethnic, politicised friends as strange as he thought me. My crazies were just too crazy. They baffled him and probably left him feeling confounded and powerless.

To the astonishment of the family and everyone who knew us, Jonty became a businessman. It was anathema to all of us. Journalist, art student, barmaid, rabbi, window cleaner, lumberjack, waitress, lecturer, shop assistant, human rights lawyer, nightclub hostess, out-of-work teacher – at some time or another one of us was one of these things, and all of them were acceptable, even normal, pursuits. But the pursuit of money was entirely strange. However, Jonty was brilliant and showed flair, eventually confounding all of us by making a success of his career and his life.

Just in case my own family wasn't large or expansive enough, I invented a whole new one to throw into the festivities: Tania and her family, a somewhat Bohemian band of gypsies. One day, when I was five, my nursery school teacher, Rosa Woolf, transcribed a conversation she had had with me about Tania. It went like this:

Rahla: When Tania and me were playing, we were pretending we heard an animal and we really did hear an animal and they were dogs. And when we were playing we asked our mom if we could dress up in her clothes because we wanted to do a play for my mother; we did *Fair Rosy*.

Rosa: Where does Tania live?

Rahla: She lives in the same world as us but on the other side. Tania's mother is Janet. Do you want to know her surname?

Rosa: Yes.

Rahla, ignoring the teacher: We're not friends any more and I thought she was on holiday. Tania's brother is called Richard. The baby's name is Anne; they live in a crabby place. The big boy puts the baby where the crabs can't eat it.

I've always considered it perfectly ordinary to have an imaginary friend. My mother says Tania and her family were the easiest people she ever entertained. Clearly they were loyal and steadfast friends, but, most importantly, they required me to entertain them. They would sit in the garden and I would put on a show for them. I would dance and prance through Broadway number after Broadway number, both bold and whimsical, and they never tired of being my captivated, captivating audience.

Sometimes Daddy took us, one at a time, to tag along with him on his Sunday ward round. As he popped in on the psychiatrically unstable, we'd wait with pretty young nurses who apparently had nothing better to do than feed us scoops of vanilla ice cream and hospital jelly.

One Sunday, Daddy and I were driving to the clinic in his dashing navy-blue Peugeot. On a busy road he suddenly heard an alarming shriek erupt from the back seat. Swerving round to look at me, he screeched to a halt as I yelled, 'Daddy, stop, you're going to crash into Tania!' On that occasion he was as mad as hell at me for nearly causing an accident, but my mother insisted it wasn't my fault, as he should have just ignored me.

Tania remained my friend for years. She had alabaster skin and golden hair cascading all the way down, down, down to her bum, and she couldn't be frightened off by oncoming traffic, nursery school or even – some of the time – laughing old men. She stuck by me, strong and bold as Queen Latifah, until I really needed her – until I went friendless and alone into the unwelcoming world of school.

After that, she and all her family vanished, never to be seen or heard from again. As I imagine did a part of me, and a part of every child, on that first day when we are marched off to school in shiny shoes, socks pulled up, teeth and faces lovingly polished, and that obstinate wayward curl combed down with water or a dollop of Mommy's hair gel. But there it is – such is the way of the world. Tania could not have walked with me down the classroom aisle, to the chair directly in front of the teacher's menacing glare any more than that obstinate curl could remain in place after first break.

Fortunately, I also had a *real* best friend, Brian. He lived across the road, and he felt more like a sibling than a friend. Brian was there all my life, like Fenster Number 6. When we were little, we weren't allowed to cross the road to one another's houses, and on some days, while waiting for an available grown-up to lead one of us across, that road felt like the forbidden staircase between downstairs and the surgery upstairs where Daddy worked all day, like the endless distance from birthday to birthday. Later the road got so narrow it seemed as if Brian's bedroom was an extension of mine, and I'd hide from my dates inside his mother's cupboards. Until one boy got smart and parked his car outside Brian's house, knowing that I couldn't survive the entire day without going over there.

By the time I was born, my mother Lviah had taken on the nickname Livicky, because my father used to serenade her, 'Livicky my wife, the joy of my life.' By then, the long tresses were long gone, and part of her no-nonsense look was a shock of short, punky, black hair. (This was before short, punky hair was a style.) She was a speech and drama teacher, and sometimes I'd make myself at home under the piano in the studio while she taught. I have a memory of her sitting in front of the fire night after night, sewing feathers onto a lilac peacock suit for me to wear in her production of *The Tempest*. I would wear that outfit day and night; I wore it until it literally fell off my body.

Livicky was small and pretty, quick as a whip and always laughing. She *loved* to laugh, and Daddy made her laugh. Quite striking with her pixie-like hair, she never wore a stitch of make-up. Naturally I always wanted a fashionable mother, one with long hair in styled flicks who wore lipliner and frothy dresses, but Livicky was utterly inept at any form of fashion, or sports for that matter.

But she was always wildly creative. Once she turned my birthday party into a 'butterfly ball'. There were Chinese lanterns in the garden and pale, shiny worms made out of meringue, with liquorice feelers. Each of my siblings did different activities with the guests, and at the end Livicky and Daddy, all dressed up, danced a waltz together. Livicky was never the old woman who lived in a shoe; she always knew precisely what to do with her myriad children.

Writing about my mother is an intimidating task, particularly given the fact that she so expressly does not want to be written about.

But this is a love story, and love stories are about lives costumed in romance and lit up by fantasy. I never took for granted the epic love my parents shared. It was always something rare and special, an inspiration, along with fairy tales and love songs.

Livicky's own mother was a great music critic and impresario who travelled the world writing reviews of music concerts and glamorously entertaining musicians. Livicky's father, serious and brilliant, had had to give up his dream career as a psychiatrist because of a hearing deficiency, becoming an ophthalmic surgeon instead. My grandparents lived in Port Elizabeth, a drowsy seaside town infamous for its windiness but famous for the friendliness of its inhabitants.

It was in that windy city that Daddy first met Livicky. At thirty-six, he was something of a confirmed bachelor, an almost pathologically bookish scholar, having pursued his studies for thirteen years. He'd grown up in Johannesburg, the metropolitan capital of South Africa, where his father had made his money in the unrefined business of motor spares.

In Livicky's family of intellectuals, wealth was considered somewhat vulgar, a thing to be discreet, if not ashamed, about. But Daddy was irresistible: tall and charming, a medical student and a marvellous athlete. Most appealing was the fame he'd achieved for being funny; it was the stuff of which aphrodisiacs are made.

Daddy went to Port Elizabeth to visit his sister and saw Livicky acting in a play. He knew. Instantly, he just knew. The next day, he took her on a date. They walked along the promenade. And she *knew*. A gust of wind swept them both off their feet. He felt the earth move. He felt the clouds come tumbling down, tumbling down. When he dropped her off at home, to her horror he failed to propose. But she saw him the following day, and the day after that. On the fourth day, finally, he proposed.

Livicky used to tell us that as soon as she looked into his blue eyes, hooded under their great bushy brows, she knew one thing was as sure as her own mortality: this was the man who would always make her laugh.

Livicky's mother, Millie, returned from a trip abroad. 'Hello, dear, what have you been up to?' she asked.

Confident as the sea is about its waves, Livicky responded: 'I got engaged!'

Millie tried to maintain her sophisticated poise. 'Oh, to whom?'

'Gerald!'

'Gerald who?'

'I don't know his surname. He's just Gerald and I love him and we're engaged to be married!'

Livicky's father, Jacob, had always barred her from the kitchen, which he'd considered too dangerous an environment for his only child. For her, it was an uninviting, boring place. With marriage imminent, Jacob phoned Gerald and requested an urgent meeting. Gerald flew nervously to Port Elizabeth, where he and Jacob walked in awkward silence on the windy promenade. Eventually, with deep regret, Jacob blurted out, 'She can't cook; she'll never cook.'

Daddy's roar of unconcerned laughter was carried by the wind over the ocean and would echo through all the days of their glorious life together.

Within three months, they were married. They basked in the glory of a hurly-burly romance for nearly forty years. Every morning of our young lives, we were woken by the alarm clock of Livicky's infectious laughter. Until I met Jason, I thought such epic romance existed only in fairy tales and under my parents' roof.

Mealtimes in our house were loving and loud, happy and gregarious events. There were always so many children and friends and lovers.

If you went to the telephone or the toilet, a sibling or a friend would sometimes hide your plate of food on your chair as a prank. But it was funny – everything was funny. Livicky laughed out loud all the time. Daddy made her laugh.

Both dominating and illuminating our small dining room was a large brass rococo clock. It was ornately decorated with birds, flowers and shells, and weighted down by two heavy, rather phallic-looking lead balances reluctantly swinging back and forth on heavy chains.

The clock tick-tocked away through all our laughter and tears, through the intimacy of all the Friday nights and the glamour of Sunday lunches, from all the great feasts to the mundane Thursday-night macaroni-and-cheese suppers. Even now I can still tick-tock myself effortlessly back in time to the witty Sunday lunches that began at noon and ended with cold soup and French loaves only at midnight.

The house was permeated with the velvety smell of cigars, as it was the late 1970s and people still smoked indoors. As always, my father effortlessly held court. Languidly the flow of anecdotes would go on, words dripping off his tongue like treacle.

'I was escorting a disturbed patient out of South Africa,' he would begin, 'home to his native Belgium, because he'd been caught under the Immorality Act.' (A time warp into past lunacy, the Immorality Act was one of the more immoral acts of the bizarre institution called apartheid. According to this law, it was illegal for a man and a woman of different races to engage in sexual relations, and the guilty white party would either be imprisoned or deported, were he or she a foreigner.) Daddy paused for effect, as the liberals around the table chuckled out loud. According to Daddy's story, it had been decided by the mental-health authorities that the emotionally disturbed patient would be safer in Belgium than in South Africa, with its immoral laws.

To ease his own passage through bureaucracy, Daddy had written an official letter on his own behalf: 'Dr Fenster is escorting a highly disturbed patient to his place of origin. Any help you can provide him with in this matter would be greatly appreciated. Signed, Dr Gerald Fenster.'

Armed with his patient, the letter and a medical kit of psychotropic paraphernalia, Daddy boarded the aeroplane, immediately administering a sleeping pill to both himself and his patient. But the patient didn't succumb fast enough. With his last resource of wakeful energy, in the brief moment just after the aircraft took off and before the pill kicked in, the patient stood up and hollered: 'We've now flown out of South Africa, and I will fuck whomever I please on this aeroplane!'

With which the great Casanova collapsed on top of my father, who was a little too out of it to notice that the seats around him were emptying in a hurry. A manicured red nail tapping urgently on his shoulder rudely woke him up. The air hostess, in a demure navy crimplene skirt and navy pillbox hat, said: 'Dr Fenster, please guard your patient at all times. He has unsettled everyone, and you can't afford to nod off on this journey.'

Thick-tongued and slurring, Daddy reassured her: 'Not to worry, he's as subdued as a lamb, fast asleep. As we should all be. Now, if you'll excuse me ...'

The air hostess returned with an irate captain. 'Dr Fenster, the man next to you is a highly disturbed and clearly dangerous individual, as is specified in the official letter of warning you're carrying. It's imperative that you do not sleep on this flight.'

All night long the highly disturbed patient slept like a lamb, and all night long the officious air hostess trotted up and down the aisle delivering polystyrene cups of bitter instant coffee to my irascible father.

Landing exhausted in Belgium, he found no family members waiting to greet the highly disturbed but drowsy patient, so he hailed a taxi and delivered the patient to his family on their farm.

Driving back into town and finally half dozing off, Daddy vaguely heard the burble of the driver through the haze of the previous night's sleeping pill. 'Isn't it a shame that they're tearing down this old farmhouse to build a highway? Now the owners are selling everything and moving away.' Alerted from his slumber by the words 'old' and 'selling', my father shouted to the driver to pull over.

There, in the rubble of a demolished Belgian farmhouse, he caught sight of a romantic dismantled clock. Suddenly convinced that he could communicate fluently in Flemish, Daddy greeted the farmer's family and asked if he could buy the clock. By way of response, they laughed at him.

Cautiously, he named a price. They threw up their hands in mock-horror. Embarrassed, he hastily raised his price. At which they threw up their hands again and all started shouting at once. Humiliated, he raised his offer considerably. At which they threw up their hands, shouted, pointed at him and laughed out loud.

At this point the taxi driver intervened, alerting my father to the fact that his Flemish wasn't up to the task, because the farmers were bargaining him down as he was bargaining them up. They were trying to explain to him that what they wanted was the price of a modern alarm clock. An outrageously unfair price was agreed upon, and they all sat down to drink yet another cup of coffee. Daddy, ever the guilty tourist, managed to slip a few dollars under his cake plate, and they all helped carry the clock, weights and all, to the taxi.

The practical difficulties involved in transporting such a clock home across the ocean didn't occur to my father until he arrived back at his hotel. He was a fabulous father, a great psychiatrist, a witty raconteur, a devoted husband and many other things, but practical he was not.

This was the hottest summer Europe had had in decades, so Daddy stripped down to shorts, flip-flops and, inexplicably, a raincoat, then packed up and shipped all his clothes and toiletries back to South Africa. The cumbersome clock he managed to wedge inside the suitcase, but not the leaden weights. So he sat down to write another official letter: 'Mr Fenster is suffering from a slipped cervical disc and must wear his weights at all times. Signed, Dr Fenster.'

Those solid lead weights were heavy, but he managed to hoist the chain over his neck and swing them on either side of his broad girth. His new 'official' letter got him out of Belgium, onto the aeroplane and into his seat. With a huge sigh of relief, he removed the weights, only to feel a familiar tapping on his shoulder. He looked up to be greeted by another crimplene skirt and navy pillbox hat. 'Mr Fenster, if Dr Fenster says you wear your weights, you wear your weights!'

The aeroplane landed in Johannesburg two hours ahead of schedule. It was 6 a.m., early June 1969. In his travelling outfit of weights, shorts, raincoat and flip-flops, Dr Fenster disembarked from the aircraft in agony. The first blast of icy wind cutting painfully into his exposed calves alerted him to the obvious. If it was the hottest summer in Europe, it stood to reason that South Africa was enduring the coldest winter in decades. The country, famous for its cruel constitution and sunny skies, was experiencing snowfalls on the Highveld – an event so extraordinary it wouldn't recur for nearly two decades.

Naturally, looking the way he did, Dr Fenster was stopped by customs officials. He was too exhausted to carry the weights for another minute, so with trembling hands he produced not the 'slipped disc' letter, but the 'extremely disturbed' one. Upon reading the letter, the Afrikaans customs official erupted with laughter, calling a colleague who resembled an ageing Truman Capote, and said, '*Kom Piet, kom kyk na hierdie maljan.*' (Come Pete, come and look at this madman.)

They escorted my father to a private room, sat him down, removed the weights and his travel pouch, wrapped him in a blanket, and handed him a plate of cheese sandwiches with the crusts cut off and a polystyrene cup of cheap coffee with heaps of extra sugar (because it is assumed that mad people are in a permanent state of shock and must be given extra sugar to soothe their frayed nerves).

From a safe distance the two customs officials sat watching the madman drink his coffee and eat his sandwiches, while outside security desperately paged the airport arrivals area. 'Calling Dr Fenster, would Dr Fenster please report to customs immediately. Your patient urgently needs your assistance, Dr Fenster.'

Cautiously and from a safe distance the officials enquired in the gentle, patronising tone reserved for irate children and madmen, 'Hey, mister, mister Fenster, what you got in your big suitcase?' In his finest Queen's English, with a deadpan expression, the madman responded, 'Oh, that's a grandfather clock,' and carried on eating his sandwich as the officials continued to study the *maljan* and security tried to page Dr Fenster.

Eventually, taking a bold step forward, the Afrikaans customs officer said, 'Hey, mister, why don't you show us your grandfather clock?' Placing his polystyrene cup of coffee on the chair in front of him, the *maljan* replied, 'Yes, indeed, I do believe I shall.' But of course the key for the lock of the suitcase was in the confiscated pouch awaiting the arrival of the elusive Dr Fenster.

It was at this point that Daddy, his coffee finished, his plate of sandwiches emptied, his body thawed and his spine mildly relieved, decided the charade was up and it was time to go home to his family.

He stood up and said, 'Now look here, there's been a misunder-standing. *I* am Dr Fenster.' At which the customs officials doubled up with laughter and the Capote lookalike said, '*Ja, en ek is Napoleon.*' (Yes, and I am Napoleon.)

Daddy managed to convince them to retrieve his pouch with his passport to prove both his identity and his sanity. Almost satisfied, the customs officials demanded to see the contents of the case. Daddy opened the case to display the clock. The official asked sarcastically, 'Why can't a psychiatrist use an ordinary wristwatch?'

Later, arriving shivering but relieved at his own front door, Daddy was barred from entry by Pnina and David, who were adding the final touches to his 'welcome-home' posters. So he waited ten min-utes in the freezing cold, with his suitcase and clock by his side. Kissing Livicky hello, he produced the clock and laid it out proudly on their bed. Livicky, pregnant with me, looked at it and said, 'I don't like it; it's too ornate and kitsch. Take it back.'

Visions of having to put the weights back on, go through customs and be bullied by the crimplened air hostess again flashed through Daddy's mind. The look of horror on his face made Livicky giggle. 'Don't worry,' she said. 'I'll learn to like it. Get some rest.'

Ironically, three months later Daddy felt a stabbing pain shoot through his spine. 'Gerald, you've got a slipped cervical disc,' his doctor said. 'I'm going to put you into traction, and you'll have to wear heavy weights.' Naturally Daddy didn't comply; he wasn't big on listening to doctors.

Family stories. It's a funny thing about life – we never understand, or at least it takes us so long to understand one another properly. I think it happens in all families: the vulnerable ones are the strong ones, the wounded ones are those who live most fearlessly, and the damaged ones are often those who live most joyously. A family becomes a person, really.

I know growing up could not have been as entirely hunky-fucken-dory as I choose to remember it. Under hypnosis on a velvet chaise longue, I'm sure I'd find layers of the usual dysfunctional stuff in my family's dynamics. It must have been unbalanced; the baby sister with so many needs must have drained some of the resources both financially and emotionally. No family sails through altogether untroubled waters, and a family with chemical disorders inevitably goes through tempests. I suspect Jonty struggled to understand why I constantly needed lifts from therapists to doctors to remedial teachers, none of whom succeeded in pacifying me. None of whom succeeded in normalising me.

And Daddy could fly into a purple rage most unexpectedly. Often I would be at the receiving end, maybe because subconsciously he saw too many similarities between us, or just because I was the most exasperating of all the children. But Gigi protected me from his anger, as she has tried to protect me all my life – from bullies in the playground, from financial blacklisting and negligent doctors, from overdoses and dinner parties I found myself incapable of hosting. She protected me from a world I often found too brittle to bear.

Family life was never dull. Pnina had lots of boyfriends. They were all drawn to her brilliance and beauty, her lush sexuality. One of the boyfriends, the smooth, sexy Conrad Cline, would take two headache pills before coming to dinner just to help him cope with the family's boisterousness. Gigi, kind and clever, brought to the noisy table her impossibly tall Dutch husband and their two perfect children, Ruth and Hannah.

One night Daddy was feeling flush because he had just won a medical legal case. Livicky wasn't aware of this, so she wasn't feeling flush at all. Daddy scraped his food across his chipped plate, saying, 'I don't much like this old plate. I've never actually liked it. I'm going to smash it. Would anybody care to join me in the ceremonial smashing of tired old plates?'

Livicky went white, knowing he was irrepressible. Under his rebel influence, we were all irrepressible. Crash! Plates were smashing one by one; all the children were laughing and throwing their plates against the dining-room wall.

I never thought of Daddy as being 'up' or 'down'. I know he was stupendous and effervescent, that he had insanely marvellous stories and that, unbelievably, they were all true. But as the Happy Potter doctor once told me, 'The well bipolars rule the world.' My father not only ruled the world, he rocked it!

Many people have an inner light – I've known people with a light so bright it dazzled, quite blinding me – but Daddy's light was rare in that it illuminated our journeys. Searching for the elusive words for phenomena that have no name, trying to make sense of it all, of the world inside my head, a world sometimes gone quite mad, thinking of him, the clock story comes back to me. Other outrageous stories crop up before me and I think of a guiding light illuminating the path, not all the way, but just enough for me to take one faltering step at a time.

Looking back now, so much older and possibly more aware, I suppose his outbursts may have been chemically induced. I imagine he had periods of mania and then sank into periods of depression. But who could have known? He masked it well.

We were all so ignorant back then. And, of course, he self-medicated with sleeping pills and diet pills and I don't really know what else. Whatever was or wasn't wrong with him, he succeeded not only in coping with the ups and downs, but in gathering our daily lives up into a joyous, outlandish celebration that transformed what could otherwise have been a rather financially stretched childhood.

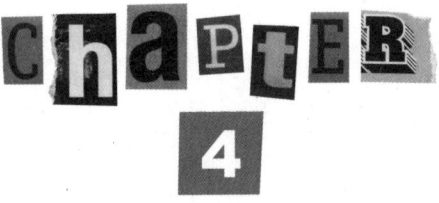

4

And then the whining schoolboy, with his satchel / And shining morning face, creeping like snail / Unwillingly to school.

— WILLIAM SHAKESPEARE, *AS YOU LIKE IT*

School was a cruel joke. Until I went to school, the enchantment of my early childhood meant that I felt confident that I was loveable and pretty and clever. My siblings and my parents contrived to maintain this illusion.

King David Primary didn't take to my hair. I often say, 'I'm not crazy, I just have curly hair.' But at six years old, I didn't have any funny things to say about my exuberant curls. Other children did. 'Chewing-gum hair' was a favourite. Also, on account of having

39

been a breech birth, I had little 'horns' on either side of my head. Because of my slanting eyes, I was called 'China eyes'. And my two front teeth were brown from cortisone medication for an ear infection I'd had in infancy. I looked like a combination of Nicholas Nickleby and the Little Match Girl.

My parents sensibly believed that what money was available should be spent on good education and medical care. School uniforms, tights included, were darned and handed down to me as the baby of the family. Everything was a little worn and damaged by the time it reached me. Pnina and Gigi were taller than me, so their hand-me-down skirts hung unflatteringly down to my ankles. Altogether I was a peculiar-looking child. King David Primary didn't take well to peculiar.

In addition to my bizarre appearance, I was dyslexic, hyperactive and generally not well adjusted. The other kids teased me mercilessly, and somehow the teachers never noticed.

When I was about seven, I was sent to Anita, a child psychologist who worked with my father. I adored her. I used to go to Anita after school and we'd talk. She told me that I was depressed. My father had recognised depression in me at an early age, but Livicky said she'd never encountered a depressed child. The mere notion of a depressed child was absurd, almost unnatural, but there I was.

Anita was a down-to-earth person, someone who had cast off the confines of her strict, right-wing family. She was five times the South African archery champion, Daddy's best friend, and an old-fashioned lesbian who wore calf-length skirts and unflattering shoes. She was precise, loving and funny. I imagine what drew her and Daddy, a child psychiatrist, to one another was their innate, instinctive understanding of children. It was Anita's tranquillity, her quiet, which got me through the rage of school.

Once a week I went to hang out with Anita. I don't remember exactly what we did. We'd talk, play, do shows; it felt safe there, even normal, surrounded by her eccentric collection of miniature books and bows and arrows. In her deep, earthy Afrikaans accent she'd tell me stories and explain things to me. It was as if we were two moles, tunnelling way, way under the ground where no one could see us. And yet sometimes it got too dark down there, because on occasion I'd hide, running across to my neighbour Brian's house, bunking from Anita, hiding from the darkness within.

One Sunday she arrived at the front door holding a grubby shoe-box with holes punctured in the lid. Inside slept a puppy – Lolly, my first dog, the first of my miniature dachshunds.

Lolly would outlive Anita. When I was nineteen, she and Daddy decided medical aid was a waste of money. Within six months he had had his first bad fall and she had cancer. She was dead within a year.

Early one morning, the house still quite silent and peaceful, I heard the clang, clang of my fathers' crutches coming up the passageway towards my bedroom. Opening the door, he had a look of shock, but said simply, with no adjectives to soften the blow, 'Anita died.' I inherited her most precious possession, an Omega De Ville watch.

After I'd been at King David for two years, all of us children, Gigi, Jonty and me, as well as my friend Brian, moved to Rosebank Primary. But I didn't fare much better there.

In the classroom, in the playground, being shoved out of the tuck-shop queue, on the school bus and in my own nervous, out-of-place skin, I was an outsider. At birthday parties, I was the uninvited. In anything related to ball skills, I had three left feet and a gammy right arm. Athletics left me inert, paralysed in terror. And,

41

being dyslexic, reading aloud had me confusing Bs with Ds and hyperventilating in fear.

I'd have been a dead loss had it not been for my one shining passion – the passion to perform, to step into the light. I knew my mark, and it was centre stage! When I danced, the music inhabited me, lifting my gyrating frame up, up and away from all this, away to a new world under a new sky, in free flight towards the beseeching light. And then I was 'Up down turn around, please don't let me hit the ground.'

In acting, I could lose myself. In other people's words, in characters leading lives entirely unrelated to my own. I was not 'just this girl', I was some kind of wonderful. I was the beautiful and the damned, the great and the glorious. I was Scott's Zelda and Kurt's Courtney.

So long as someone was watching me, I could twirl around on Shirley Temple's *Good Ship Lollipop*, a lovely trip to the candy shop. In a shredded velvet leotard, fishnet tights and with a fake beauty spot, life was a *Cabaret*, old chum, and I loved a cabareeeet! With a blonde wig and thrift-store red dress I wanted to be loved by you, just you, nobody else but you. I couldn't aspire to fill the desire to anything higher than to make you my own, boop-boop-a-doop! And of course, with a long, long cigarette and a deep, deep voice, I was just an old-fashioned girl with an old-fashioned mind, not sophisticated, just the plain and simple kind. I liked the old-fashioned flowers, violets were for me, have them made in diamonds by the man at Tiffany.

And that was part of the repertoire I developed before I turned eight. I'm tone-deaf. I can't sing for toffee. But the lack of any talent didn't dampen my astonishing, unfounded confidence.

It was the gift God had given me to get through what would have been an otherwise talentless life. It was the moment within the moment, the girl within the girl, the greatest escape since *The Thomas Crown Affair*.

It was at Rosebank Primary that I met Adam Levin. All the kids in Standard 4 were having a *Xanadu* party. They were dressing up and going to see the movie, starring Olivia Newton-John, after which they'd have lunch at Steers and go roller skating on the roof of the Hyde Park shopping centre. I was the only one not invited. Adam Levin said that if they didn't invite me, he wouldn't go. In Standard 4, you couldn't have a party without Adam. You still can't.

For the occasion, I wanted a pastel-coloured pantsuit elasticised at the waist with spaghetti straps, a look that was all the rage. My parents considered this to be out of the question. On the day of the party, I went to Pnina's place to dress. A well-adjusted student, she was mildly stoned and going through a 'hippie–ethnic' phase. She blow-dried my hair straight and dressed me in a deep-purple, embroidered Indian dress with a broad tasselled belt covered in tiny mirrors. I was the only girl at the party wearing a skirt, and that was just another in a long line of misplaced outfits. Still, I enjoyed the party and the movie so much that when I got a kitten, I called it Xanadu.

Even after four years I couldn't adjust and settle down at Rose-bank Primary. The only other choices were for me to attend a remedial school or a convent. My parents wisely decided that if I went to a remedial school, I would consider myself stupid for the rest of my life, so we tried a convent. In the beginning I felt like a character in a fifties musical. Maybe a little like a young Julie Andrews. I loved the uniform and the old Victorian building with its promise of ghosts. The words of The Lord's Prayer were lovely, and the sight of shrivelled nuns running rosaries through their veined hands struck me as madly exotic and romantic.

Around this time (I guess I must have been about thirteen) I developed a wild crush on a friend of my grandmother's. Audrey was an Irish rose, ever so pretty and lyrical, with the dainty skip of a cake ballerina. A crystal chandelier dominated her lounge; a picture of me smiling among roses with my hair unusually tidy dominated her bedroom. Best of all, Audrey had Christmas.

Audrey celebrated Christmas in a big way – the angel smiling resplendently out at the world from atop a ten-foot tree. The lights winking on and off, the kisses under the mistletoe, the golden crackers banging and bursting open to reveal trinkets, bonbons and other delights. The turkey, and the dessert that dramatically caught fire. The stuffed stockings on the mantelpiece, the cake and the candy, the mountains of gifts. She even let me taste the yucky French champagne with bubbles that burst forth and tingled on my tongue.

As a nice Jewish girl I thought I'd died and gone to heaven. Christmas was paradise! This was love! This was *The Nutcracker Suite*, and I was poised perfectly in an arabesque on top of a fluffy white world.

I observed Audrey's every move and hung on her every word. When the time came for me to be schlepped over to the convent, I was ever so cool with that, because Audrey had been a nun. She told me, 'I joined the convent in the fifties, when the girls wore long, full skirts, and when I came out into the world I was met by girls in minis.' She was entirely unaware of my tattiness or my tardiness, and I loved her for it.

Then, one morning, after school had broken up, Livicky came into my bedroom, pulled open the pale-blue curtains and sat gently on my bed. 'Darling, I've got some awful news, and I'm just so terribly sorry for you,' she said. 'It's a dreadful fact of life that the only thing we know for certain is that one day we will die. Last night, out of the blue, Audrey got a headache. She was rushed to hospital, and they found she had a tumour. It was all quite sudden. She didn't suffer. I'm so sorry my baby, your Audrey died.'

Boom. I went off the rails, maybe even barking bloody mad. Continued behaving strangely, getting more ostracised. Bunking, forging my father's signature and writing fake sick notes. I started smoking and swearing at the Irish nuns. I tried to climb out the window of a maths class and got stuck, halfway inside the tedium of Sister Anthony Joseph's subtractions and halfway outside, in the plush lawns of freedom. Things rapidly spiralled out of control.

The Mother Superior sent me home with a bad report card, documenting not only my floundering academics, but my aggressive approach to the system. My parents were disappointed – again. A born drama queen, and wanting them to stop being cross with me, I did the most dramatic thing a thirteen-year-old could do in 1982. I swallowed a box of Ritalin.

This was the first of my unsuccessful suicide attempts. I don't know if I was actually thinking 'death' so much as 'out, out, help, get me out of here', desperate to escape a situation that felt overwhelming, unbearable.

I remember the gloom of the Johannesburg hospital very well. I remember the guilt as I watched Daddy, usually so much larger than life, getting smaller and smaller as he walked away dejectedly down the corridor. I remember being terribly embarrassed as the handsome medical students arrived to stare into my eyes, fully dilated from the Ritalin.

And then, oddly, I remember being concerned about a baby lizard I'd caught the afternoon of the incident. It had lost its tail, and I assumed that without my nurturing presence it would die. So I'd trapped the poor thing in a matchbox, punched in holes so that it could breathe, and given it a blade of grass for company. As I lay in hospital, my guilt intensified, and I was convinced that the lizard would surely die.

I couldn't sleep all night. The following morning a state psychiatrist came to sit next to me and told me that everything would be fine. He explained that I hadn't really wanted to die; the overdose had just been a cry for help. Content with that theory, I agreed with him. I liked the ring of the phrase 'cry for help'. I felt horribly embarrassed and just wanted to go home. Livicky and Pnina came to collect me and took me to the Rosebank Hotel for breakfast, a big treat. When I got home, the lizard was gone.

By this time I knew that I would never excel at school. I wasn't fitting in and I couldn't slip out of the system unnoticed. I started to realise how glamorous rebellion would be. Most children risk an awful lot when they rebel. I had nothing to lose. Already, it seemed, the adults disapproved of me.

At fourteen, my convent career in tatters behind me, I moved to Woodmead, a particularly socially aware and politicised school. It was one of few multiracial schools in apartheid South Africa, attended by the children of many left-wing political leaders.

My parents had always been politically conscious and kept us informed about what was happening around us. Apartheid affected even those of us who were cushioned from the injustice. There were kids who went missing from school. A policeman raped a friend of mine. The police raided our school parties. They arrived regularly looking to arrest our geography teacher, a conscientious objector who refused to do army service for the apartheid government. It was comical watching Mr van Zyl, with his long hippie beard and corduroy pants, running through the classrooms to escape the police. School was radical, it was wild. On principle I refused to concentrate during the few classes I attended and did not do any homework.

I felt pent-up anger and developed ingeniously inappropriate ways of expressing it. Never underestimate the power of not caring. One day a girl came and sat next to me on the bus. She said, 'I want to sit next to you, because the boys come and sit with you.' That day, she introduced a whole new world to me. I realised to my delight that, while the teachers would always loathe me, my days of being 'the unpopular girl' were over. The days of being belittled and bullied were behind me, because now I had boys. In her early teens, nothing gets a girl as far as boys do – not good grades, not fancy clothes, not even extra pocket money.

Although I floundered academically, I excelled at boys, drama and original schemes for bunking school. And at getting motherlessly stoned. Class was dull, but there was a river at the bottom of the school property where a bunch of teenagers used to roll and smoke joints. Nothing dull about that. Boy, did we laugh. Something as innocuous as the sight of a friend's face or a pencil was enough to have us in fits. We got into deep debates about politics and human rights, and we danced and sang a lot too.

We didn't get stoned only at school. We got stoned in super-markets, at the movies, at parties and at one another's houses, but dagga was it. I never met anyone who tried anything stronger. Nowadays the drug scene is more sinister.

Not surprisingly, I failed twice, so by the time I should have been matriculating and ready to leave school, I still had another two years to go. I had no intention of doing those two years and fluctuated between ambitions of becoming a hairdresser and a famous actress. Legally, I wasn't allowed to leave school till I'd completed Standard 8. By the time I was allowed to leave, I wanted to leave the country, too. And, with barely a Standard 8, university wasn't opening its loving academic arms to me.

The most accessible place for a nice Jewish girl like me was Israel.

My parents dreamt that the family would follow me there. It was decided: I was to spend six months in a kibbutz learning Hebrew in a sheltered environment, after which I could venture out into the cities. As it transpired, I think the Cape Flats would have provided me with a more sheltered environment.

Before leaving South Africa, I set about the task of losing my virginity. I marked my target, waited for the night of my eighteenth birthday and got done with the deed. Mission accomplished, I set off on my awfully big adventure.

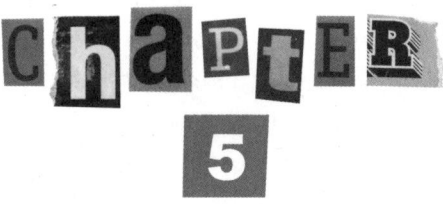

CHAPTER 5

An awfully small, awfully silly adventure

Israel — for such a small country it sure packs some diversity. My time there was pretty weird. A couple of years ago, I was walking into a theatre in Cape Town when a girl came up to me and said, 'Aren't you Rahla? I remember sitting in your flat in Israel, having my first joint. I stared at a poster of Marilyn Monroe and thought, oh my God, I'm really stoned.'

I wondered about this information. Did I really have a flat in Israel? Did I have visitors, presumably friends? What happened to the Marilyn Monroe poster? I looked for the girl after the show, but she was gone. She'd appeared to be a straightforward, lovely girl with no reason to lie. I thought, had I been established enough as a human being to be a bad influence back then? Did I have a life in

Israel? Not one photograph exists of my time there, and I'd always assumed this was because I'd had no friends to take any.

I departed for Israel on a high. It had been a wonderful summer. I'd been laughing and dancing and flirting and partying my curly head off. Without my virginity, I considered myself a sophisticated woman. Best of all, school was behind me. Forever.

I wore a denim Levi jacket that Jonty had brought back from America (those were the days of trade sanctions against South Africa, so anything remotely 'cool' came from abroad). Brand-new skin-tight denims followed my every perfect skinny curve, and the Reebok sneakers Daddy had bought me gave additional spring to my step. Waving goodbye were my family, my friend Brian and a boyfriend who looked rather like a Labrador. I embarked on my first international flight, singing along with the Pretenders, 'I'm walking on sunshine ...' The world seemed a simple place. I was wild with excitement and joy.

In the beginning it was fun living in Israel. Cold, but fun. Boys liked me, and one night I had so much to drink that I got alcohol poisoning, which was considered a cool thing to happen. I mopped floors and wiped dirty tables after dinner. The *kibbutzniks* used to ask the white South Africans how many 'slaves' we had. All South Africans were automatically assumed to be racist, bad people, this being at the height of apartheid.

I found the *kibbutzniks* a bit hard and ruthless. The men had a system of rating new volunteers. They picked out whom they considered to be the three best-looking girls, and those girls had it easy. What none of the dumb volunteers took into account was the fact that there were new volunteers coming in from all over the world on a constant basis, and the truth was that they were all better looking when they arrived than they were after a couple of weeks of waking up at the crack of dawn, eating too much bread and feeling homesick.

The kibbutz was situated right at the sea. On bitterly cold evenings we would run across the beach to the ancient ruins of Caesarea. Without knowing much about the Bible, I could stand among the ruins under a full moon and get carried away by the melodrama of the ancient tales, believing in the misogynistic, violent stories I'd laughed off all my life.

One night I was having coffee with a friend when the owner of the restaurant approached us for a chat. He bought us a couple of drinks. He was handsome, stylish and witty, but what appealed to my overinflated vanity most was his flattery. My friend was quick to notice that he was wearing expensive shoes. This, she explained, was a good sign.

At dawn I found myself walking back to the kibbutz on sunshine. The following evening, after wiping the dirty dinner tables, we went back, this time with more friends, who were sick of the fresh, wholesome kibbutz food. We all enjoyed a free meal and admired the natty shoes.

It became a habit to hang out at this restaurant with this man, Moshe, who was willing to pay for everything. Because of the luxuries I could so effortlessly procure from my older 'boyfriend', I became really popular among the volunteers on the kibbutz. Moshe proudly introduced me to his 'brothers and nephews', none of whom was actually related to him, as Moshe explained. They worked for him and were utterly loyal to him, and if ever I needed anything, anything at all, his 'brothers and nephews' would see to it for me.

Moshe decided that kibbutz food wasn't good enough for me, so every day he'd send his 'relatives' round to the front gate to deliver plates of food from the restaurant. One day they'd drive up in an old station wagon, the following day in a shiny new Mercedes-Benz. I considered none of this irregular, but it was around this time that I became distinctly unpopular with the kibbutz authorities.

Although Moshe owned most of the nightclubs in the area, he never seemed to do any work. He read the paper to check how his 'shares' were doing, held meetings with his 'relatives' and played an awful lot of tennis. We'd go clubbing in a nearby town and Moshe would pay for my milkshakes in Swiss francs. Still, none of this struck me as unusual.

One day, a policeman came to the kibbutz asking for me. When I told Moshe about the visit he was furious, saying that the policeman had spotted me walking about in Caesarea and that he claimed to be in love with me. This was unacceptable behaviour, and one of the 'nephews' would have to sort him out. The following day my friend and I bumped into the policeman, who looked at us sheepishly. He had a black eye and bore other signs of a beating.

Belatedly, I started to recall the gangster movies I'd watched, but as soon as I put the pieces together, I shrugged them off as preposterous. This was the stuff of American cinema, and I'd been raised on a diet of European art films. Then the head of the kibbutz called me into his office to explain that the men I was hanging out with were scumbags. They were the local mafia and not suitable companions for a nice Jewish girl from South Africa.

In South Africa I'd rebelled against conformity, the insanity of apartheid and the horror of school. But I had never really had much need to rebel against my family, so I remained a protected child. Out there in the land of milk and honey, rebellion left me pretty much alone and adrift. I became miserable and put on weight. It wasn't long before loose dresses replaced my stretch denims.

The kibbutz could tolerate all manner of things, but it seemed to me that a girl getting fat was going against some ideological responsibility. I decided the best thing was to leave and go to Jerusalem, where nobody knew me.

In Jerusalem, I worked as a char cleaning apartments, a job for which I had no aptitude. One day my boss explained to me that my practice of sweeping dust under the sofa along with a pile of dirty clothes didn't really work for him. But he added that he and his children loved having me around and that he would like me to stay on for a nominal fee, with meals provided. I did.

He introduced me to his friend Gingi. Gingi came not a minute too soon. He was completely besotted with me and had no problem with an extra kilogram here or there. Gingi was in the unglamorous business of vegetable importing. All in all, he was not a terribly glamorous man.

In all the months I'd been in Israel, I'd managed, at every available opportunity, to maintain something of a sense of luxury by going to the sumptuous King David Hotel, where I'd pretend to be a guest. I'd swan around using the pool and the gym and pilfering everything from toilet paper to tea bags.

One day Gingi bought me a new dress and we made a fancy dinner for the manager of the King David Hotel, because Gingi desperately wanted to win the contract to supply the hotel with fresh produce. It was a great occasion. I painted my nails and got sparkly, animated, slightly tipsy and totally turvey. The more tippled I got, the more confident I became until, over dessert, in a drunken stupor, I blurted out to the guest of honour, 'I hope you get a good deal out of Gingi, because I must owe the King David Hotel a fucking fortune.' I told everyone at the table all of my tricks, and in my drunken daze I mistook their silence for amusement.

That night Gingi drove his car out of the trendy centre of Jerusalem in silence. The white lines in the middle of the road made me think of an airport runway warning of an ominous banishment. A couple of times I made feeble attempts at conversation.

Rahla: Wasn't Allon's wife wearing an odd dress?

Gingi: *Silence.*

Rahla: Do you think they have a good marriage, Allon and his wife?

Gingi: *Silence.*

Rahla: I thought the manager of the hotel seemed to have a great sense of humour, didn't he?

Gingi: *Silence.*

Rahla: The dessert was wicked.

Gingi: *Silence.*

We stared out at the white lines ahead. As the countryside became more remote and desolate, an olive tree or two appeared in a feeble attempt to break the miserable tedium. After a silence as long as Rapunzel's hair, the car finally idled impatiently at my front door.

Rahla: All in all, I think the evening was a success.

Gingi: Goodnight, Rahla. Go inside and sleep it off.

Watching the car speed off into the moonless night, its headlights illuminating the road markings, I recalled something I'd once read: 'There's nothing in the middle of the road but a yellow line and dead armadillos.' What was I? The yellow line, the dead armadillo or the middle of the road? Who would know? The quote was out of context, and so was I.

That night, when Gingi dropped me home, he dropped me. As devastated as I was to lose him, a surprise the following day perked me up. Returning home from my work at the laundromat, I found on my bed a huge basket wrapped in cellophane with a blue bow. Inside, compliments of the King David Hotel, were towels, a bathrobe, stationery, vouchers for the gym and pool, and cosmetics. Evidently, the manager did have a sense of humour. It was a fabulous and generous gesture, but I missed Gingi already and felt lonely.

After this incident, I felt too embarrassed to go back to the hotel. In fact, I was too embarrassed to go anywhere. The streets were harsh and the people abrupt. I ate a lot of falafels and chocolates. At the time I lived on the outskirts of Jerusalem with a woman who was an alcoholic. In order to pay the rent, I'd look after her children, a boy and a brave little girl who was paralysed from the waist down. For a while I taught drama at the little girl's school. I even managed to muster up something of a school concert. But before long I became too nervous to go to the school regularly.

I started to long for the African sun, for African music and the vibrant contrasting colours that were home, for the warmth of the people, for the summer streets I'd jogged along with my sisters.

Israel was not an adventure at all; it immobilised me. The chaos and noise silenced and frightened me. My lack of coping skills terrified me. People around me were preoccupied with the harrowing task of survival in a tough country. They didn't have time for the fears of a small, overstuffed Jewish girl from the tip of Africa.

In a super-sized tracksuit, humming a very different, disappointed song, I boarded an aeroplane for home.

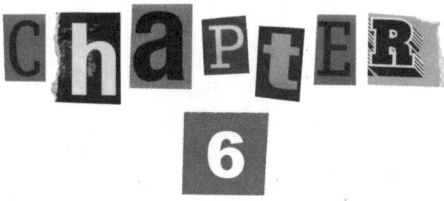

CHAPTER 6

My silent knight

I met Jason in the spring, which brings with it the smell of jasmine. Sexy, sexy world. I hadn't yet been taught to identify the symptoms, but that spring I was manic: too thin, a wild card, creative, flamboyant, and quick as a whip. In each direction I turned there were men and boys, so many men, phones ringing, doors opening, flowers being delivered, eyes glancing appraisingly.

I had no time to stop and look. I was in free flight, a glimmering, dazzling Concorde. Everyone was of interest, and yet no one was of interest for more than a brief space of time. I couldn't concentrate on anything or anyone for long. I was the incarnation, the epitome of the MTV generation with my short attention span. Glossy lips, short skirt, I moved too fast, frenetic, frenetic, weekend, Friday night,

Crowded House concert, crowded mood, crowded heart. Too many men, too many boys, all wanting something from me, wanting me.

Out there in the wilderness, we weren't real people. I was hanging out with rich kids and had momentarily mistaken myself for one of them. I seemed to know everybody at the club. I waved at someone. My ex-boyfriend glanced at me warningly, imploringly, with a sense of ownership. Christ, I'd broken up with him nearly a year ago – how did he sustain this sense of entitlement? It must have been me, feeding it, needing it. Silly me. Silly boy. Silly spring.

I went into the powder room. It smelt of cocaine. A girl I used to waitress with offered me a line. I declined; offered her my scarlet Chanel lipstick. She declined. Such are the rituals. We both looked in the mirror, not at ourselves but at one another. Checking one another out. I reminded myself of my manners and the time, said goodbye, kiss-kissed the air next to her face. Must get together. Like hell. She went on to do another line.

I stepped outside the toilet. It was noisy. I was noisy. I wanted everything, and I wanted so much that I didn't know what I wanted. I wanted sushi, fast cars, smooches under lamp posts and dances under the full moon. I wanted designer jeans. I wanted all things sparkly, spangled and labelled. All things bright and beautiful. I want, I want, I want. Inside, I was chaos.

Glancing over the crowd, my eye fell on the back of a boy with long hair, sitting at the bar. And there he was, my silent knight; all was calm. All was quiet. I couldn't make out his features, but I forgot the party, the time and the world. I approached and he turned as if he were expecting to find me there. He introduced himself, and everyone else in the room, in the world, vanished.

When I met Jason, I was twenty-four, still coming out of an anorexic phase and definitely manic. He thought this was fantastic. Mania can be very sexy. One acquires a certain glow.

I'd often heard of Jason X, who went to school with my ex-boyfriend. There was excitement in the stories about him, not unlike those that surrounded my father. I'd recently heard of something he'd done in kindness, and wanted to tell him he was a *mensch*, a good person. I'd heard that he'd come home for vacation from New York, where he was at film school. I'd heard how he'd blocked off a road in New York to make an extraordinary student film.

I've always loved movies. My family is cinematic. It's a language I've always understood. So the stories of this talented New York film student completed a romantic picture in my mind of a stoned teenager, capable of kindness, who was into cinema. He had to be arty and interesting. Plus, he was out there in the big wide world – altogether the stuff of aphrodisiacs.

I believe in love at first sight. Maybe it's history we have from previous lifetimes. We look at a person and there's a familiarity and a safety that gives us the security to feel excited. Jason is an old soul. I know I must nurture each second I have with him in this life, because I'm sure he's on his last lifetime, he's so evolved.

That night he was sitting at the bar, sexy and outlandish, laughing, and he had long curly hair and both ears pierced before it was fashionable. I was drawn to his aura. 'I felt the earth move under my feet, I felt the sky come tumbling down, tumbling down …'

We talked religion, politics and family baggage. We had a circle of light around us so strong that it prevented anyone else from coming near us. In bed later that night I told myself, 'My whole life has changed. I've met this boy.'

Entering a relationship required labour and faith, but with Jason I had a certain sense of freedom. I knew everything would be all right. I knew we were destined to grow old together. Not that there weren't obstacles – Jason being one of them. I didn't care. I was so confident that this love was bigger than us two silly mortals and our silly whims of the day. It was preordained. It was our not-to-be-thwarted destiny.

On our first date (which I set up), Jason told me the truth: he was never getting married and definitely never having children. He was upfront about the fact that he didn't want to get involved in a relationship. He felt he didn't have the emotional capacity. He could only just manage a one-night stand. I said that was cool. We consummated our relationship in a room at the Rosebank Hotel.

The next morning he drove around the block five times before dropping me off at home, because he knew that he would never see me again. He always says that I am the longest one-night stand he has ever had. And here we are, fifteen years later, still standing.

In the Jewish religion, there's a legend that goes as follows: before we are born, our soul is divided into two. The two halves are flung out across the universe, and we spend our lives searching for our other, lost half. This other half is known as your *bashert*, or soulmate. Some people never find their *bashert*. When you do, he or she is instantly recognisable to you.

At the beginning of our relationship, I told Jason, 'I'll take on the world for you, but I'll never take you on,' and that's how it is. There were times when I felt as though I had to fight the world to be with him. But never, never him. Nothing in this life surpasses the miracle of the discovery of another human being. Nothing is more precious.

Jason has cocooned me and protected me. And perhaps, in my funny way, I've protected him. He's protected me from myself, but never from joy. Always he's let the sun shine in, and with him I've blossomed. My father used to tell the Chinese fable of an old man who said to a peach tree, 'Speak to me of love,' and the peach tree blossomed. I've blossomed. The right kind of love makes us shine and gives us a safe house from whence we can go and explore the world, secure in the knowledge that the house of love stands.

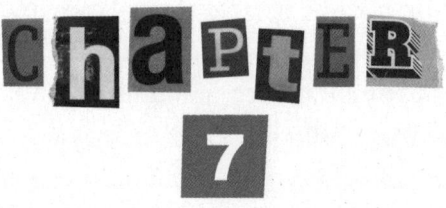

Chapter 7

What dreams may come

Families and children. I've been broody just about my entire life.

There's a part of me, an aspect of my personality, that could have ended up popping out of school, getting an inconsequential job in advertising, marrying an inconsequential man, moving into an inconsequential house. In my very early twenties I would have got down to the extremely consequential and relevant task of reproduction. In all likelihood it would have ended in tears and possibly divorce. But that's not the way it was meant to be.

What I'm saying is that I'm a born mother. I've known people who are born writers but become copywriters in advertising agencies, born artists who work in construction companies, actors who become teachers and doctors who become lawyers. Maybe doing what we dream of doing, what God intended us to do, is just a luxury, or even a great fluke. It's a shame that so many of us aren't doing what we believe we should be doing.

For years I enjoyed nurturing and teaching other people's children. Teaching is a God-given gift, one I relished. I think I did it with such devotion because it incorporated aspects of my own life's work. Perhaps a modern woman, a Virginia Slims 'we've come a long way baby' woman, ought to have a higher calling, a bigger, more ambitious dream than motherhood, but there it is. What I want, what I have always wanted, is to be someone's mother – and I can't make that dream come true. I can't seem to manifest that happiness. Maybe I've sabotaged it.

During the 'not-eating phase' of my first manic episode, my periods stopped. Ignorant youth that I was, I didn't know or particularly care what had caused this anatomical mishap. I did the maths: no boyfriend + no baby = not a care in the world.

Many years later, after a number of manic episodes and only a few periods in between, a gynaecologist explained that in all likelihood I didn't need contraception; that, having had anorexia, reproduction would probably be difficult for me. Fanfuckentastic!

When I was about twenty-four and had just met Jason, I remember lying in the bath, my toes playing with the chain hanging from the plug, fretting and crying because I wasn't getting pregnant. But it didn't matter too much, so we continued enjoying unprotected sex. (On our second date, when Jason told me he was never getting married and definitely never having children, I knew my gynaecological problems certainly weren't going to be a deal-breaker.)

Once correctly diagnosed and medicated, my body seemed to right itself. Give or take the odd kilogram here or there, my weight stabilised and my periods normalised. But perfect, pure little beings cannot be conceived or grow in a uterus pumped full of a cocktail of mood stabilisers, anti-epileptics, antidepressants, tranquillisers and sleeping pills. Likewise, precariously balanced potential mothers can't risk going off those drugs to make babies. I worried, wept, complained, bargained and fretted for weeks, which became months, which became years.

Maybe fantasies are born out of desperation. When life has consistently failed us, our embittered, disappointed minds manifest the fantasy in a desperate last bid to protect us from mediocrity and utter cynicism. And in our fantasies, because we are imagining and not actually wishing, not asking for anything, we're allowed to make our dreams as outlandish as we please. And so it was that when I'd had my empty, barren womb smashed up against reality for too many years, the idea of Tallulah, my fantasy child, was born.

She gazes up at me through the wondrous big brown eyes she inherited from her father, Jason. I find myself wondering how much she remembers of the other world before she was our little girl, commanding the full attention of our lives. Her pearly face is framed with crazy black curls she inherited from her mother – me. Some days it seems I have to catch her mid-flight, kicking and cavorting, if I'm to get a comb through those wayward, tangled locks. How am I to explain to a frantically busy four-year-old that there's an unpleasantly fine line between the charm of a defined curl and an unappealing banshee frizz? I want her neatly formed ringlets to protect her from the teasing, taunting and victimisation that plagued my own childhood.

She pirouettes through people, like a fairy apparition. The frayed hems of her long skirt trail behind her, and I pin intricately beaded fairy wings to the back of her frocks daily, as instructed. Always she carries a sense of theatre, of *Narnia* and *The Nutcracker Suite*. She seems to step into the light. I can see her aura, silvery and ancient as the moon.

She loves to dress up, loves to wriggle, to disrupt me and play with my crooked toes when I try to write. Most of all, she loves to come onto the film set and watch her father directing movies. She knows the truth about her father, that he is a magician. Sometimes when things are not too hectic, he lets her take a peek through the viewfinder to see the spells he is making.

Often I wish she didn't have to come on set alone. I wish she weren't an only child, but we always knew that, medically, we could go through only one pregnancy. All is well in the world, God is in his universe and we are all fulfilled and blissfully happy.

It's a funny-bunny, crazy-daisy world we've created, the three of us. I wonder if she orchestrated it herself. I picture her in heaven, sitting on an old brown leather suitcase surrounded by other unborn souls. God marches in, the register of humanity in his hand. In a gentle voice, he asks, 'Which of you would like a life less ordinary in Cape Town, South Africa? Your father makes moving pictures that are so sad and beautiful, they can make strangers cry. He works very hard, but he's kind and funny. He'll protect and care for you, as he has for his wife, your mother.

'Your mother,' continues God, 'has a huge capacity for love, but sometimes she's too happy and sometimes she's too sad. Sometimes she wants too much life, and some days she wants too much to die. She gets a crying germ, a germ of wings and a germ of crazies. Your father had a brother who had the same kind of waywardness in his being. I'm afraid there's a chance, if you go to this family, that you will inherit it.'

Quick as a flash, Tallulah flings up her hand eagerly, as is her way, and demands, 'If I'm their child, will I be able to dance?' God laughs and says, 'Yes, indeed my child, lots of dancing, lots of laughter and plenty of confusion. Confusion and hard work with feelings, an abundance of feelings.' And Tallulah just about leaps off her chair in excitement; she chooses unpredictable moods, art and summers in the sun, rainbows dancing over her shadow in winter.

Of course Tallulah didn't really exist. She wasn't even conceived, let alone born. But we could dream, couldn't we?

For a couple of years she was an absolute nonsense, pie-in-the-sky dream. Later, after spending time, tears and money at two fertility clinics, she became a biological factor. Frozen, I imagined her in a kindergarten of sorts in the Cape Fertility Clinic. I wondered with my friends if we couldn't bring her home, maybe just on weekends, and keep her in a silver ice bucket with a bottle of Moët.

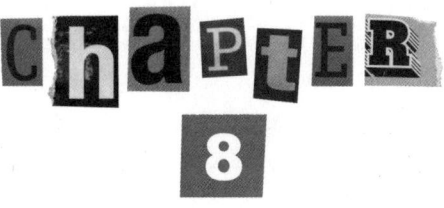

CHAPTER 8

Lights, camera, action

Forty years ago, Livicky said to my father, 'Darling, I'm in labour.' After all, it was her fifth time, and she could tell the signs. He looked at his watch and replied, 'If we leave now, we'll just make a movie.' And so it was that Livicky heavy-breathed through the adverts and the feature, a thriller starring Jean-Paul Belmondo. Then they made it down the road to the hospital, where I was born. Fortunately, I'm the kind of girl who never comes early.

When I was a child, my parents considered it appropriate to sneak me into art-house movies, where I failed to appreciate Fellini, and all five of us children used to lie on David's bed watching Charlie Chaplin projected onto the ceiling. Later, as a rebellious teen, I'd curl up on the cinema chair and get swept away by the lives of the characters on screen, munching popcorn and pitying my peers who were at school getting a mundane education.

As I so loved movies, I inevitably wanted to be involved in making them. I left school to become a movie star — or that's what I thought at the time. But a movie set is far from bipolar friendly. The hours are lunacy and the chaos unending. Film people are insane most of the time. It's a crazy industry; a relentless, unforgiving medium.

The role of artists is to move us from feeling here to feeling there. To do this, painters add colour, musicians add melody, writers words. But filmmakers, well, they add the whole bloody catastrophe — lights, camera, action!

The process detaches everyone from the rules that govern life. Fundamental rules, like eating breakfast in the morning and supper in the evening. Like working in the day and sleeping at night. Often films are shot on location so that people are physically removed from their homes and family. A new morality takes hold. Those who back home meditate and do yoga daily, change on set. I guess it's the only way to make a movie: for the duration of shooting, filmmakers are compelled to remain impervious to the norms of society. The chaos is the only constant.

Then along I came — the director's girlfriend, eventually wife and general hanger-on — into this chaotic world with my lifestyle rituals, my 'I have to be in bed by ten; I need exercise every second day; no thanks, I can't drink alcohol; I wake at precisely the same time each day, so could you please not disturb me.' I used to get homesick and miss my *tschatskes*, my calendar on the kitchen wall. I missed walking down to the local deli with the dogs and buying organic groceries for two. I missed ordering pizza on a Monday night.

I wouldn't change it — I wanted to stand by my man — but being on location with a film crew disorientated me. I used to get whacked, physically and emotionally. The intense creativity on set was thrilling, but not sleeping was unsettling. After a string of late nights my body got a bit manic (yeehah, let's go shopping!) or it got depressed (let's hide under the pillows and wish we were dead). And when this happened, Jason couldn't hold my hand – he was making a movie.

Most of the time I wasn't too sure who I was. Sometimes I'd feel completely detached from my life, from Jason and from everything I held dear. At times I was deeply proud of the film he was making, and at other times alienated by the source of my pride. I'd imagine that I was irritating Jason, that he was running away from me. Then he'd tell me to go back home to Cape Town, and I'd think he was trying to get rid of me. But it was just because he could see the signs of trouble – the shadows under my eyes, the frayed nerves and shaky responses.

Sometimes, just when I thought I'd die of exhaustion and cry in front of the crew, he'd yell 'Cuuuuuut!' and turn to say something like, 'Hey, gorgeous, wanna come home with me?' Then the sun would come out and I'd blossom.

Every emotion is blown up larger than life and intensified by the eye of the camera lens and the volatile atmosphere of the film set. It's a theatrical hothouse. But there exists a truth about people working on a film: in order to achieve something authentic on screen, the cast and crew have to be exposed during the filmmaking process. Maybe everyone is vulnerable from exhaustion, but people's emotions are raw and honest.

Amidst the mayhem I'd find that the creative energy fed me. This creative work – drama transformed into celluloid – was what we'd dreamt of, and we claimed it as our own. Every day we had on set was a gift to be treasured, because we never knew when the next opportunity was going to present itself. It was a bit like being stable; I just had to hold on tight and enjoy it.

Jason used to say he needed me to be by him because I was his safe house. One night, on set, he was standing on top of a bridge rigged up in midair with a loudspeaker in his hand. I called, 'Bye!' and he shouted back without hesitation, 'No, don't go! I'll jump!' Everyone laughed and said how romantic we were. To my sensible friends, this veered close to a dangerously codependent relationship. But for me, our relationship is the greatest achievement of love possible in a lifetime. It's a life's work. And, if we're happy, well, what's so bad about being codependent? We need one another, we totally depend on one another, and we always have.

One Sunday morning, while Jason was shooting a movie, I drove through the deserted streets of downtown Johannesburg. Everything was grim and dirty. Then, as I approached the set, I saw honey wagons and trucks and trailers and gesticulating crew members shouting orders over walkie-talkies, and suddenly the magic was there. A carnival of colour and life started up. Confetti, drums, singing floats and extras. My goodness, all the extras milling around in turbans and tutus and headdresses and hats. Body-painted, fire-eating, elongated green men walking on stilts, towering above us all, fluid gyrating bodies, undulating pink pelvises, purple tights shimmying – the dusty ground literally throbbed beneath them.

Each one, actor or extra, was an illuminated superstar and had been at it since 4.30 a.m. As the day progressed, they started to look frayed at the edges; they'd pause for breath, lean against trailers, draw long and hard on their cigarettes. They ate copious amounts of the cheap candy being passed around and fell about the set sleepily. Then the assistant director, or AD, hollered into the microphone, which was like an extra appendage, an extension of her body: 'Fun, fun, fun; remember, you're all having *fun!*' With which all the extras leapt up, swallowed their candy, stomped out their cigarettes and climbed up onto their stilts. They swirled around and smiled, smiled, smiled into … 'A-a-a-a-a-ction!'

It was a magical collaboration. I think that each time a movie is made, the process takes a piece out of everyone's psyche, and all the pieces are pooled together to make the movie. It's a breathtaking carnival, making something epic from nothing. Somewhere a teenager will escape from the drabness of algebra into that carnival.

Making a film is a bit like bipolar disorder – nothing happens in moderation. There are addictive days, days of creative highs, moments of total despair and periods of tension. But in the end, it's bigger than any one individual, and you just have to surrender to the process.

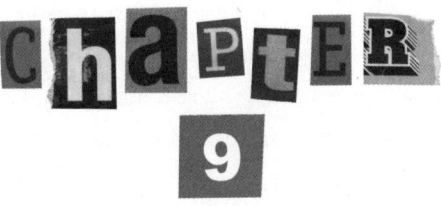

CHAPTER 9

Whenever I felt frustrated as a child, I remember 'scratching myself'. I don't really know why. Maybe it was in response to teachers talking to me harshly or my not managing homework, a kind of light relief from feelings of guilt or inadequacy. Maybe it was out of boredom, as if once I'd started I couldn't stop. I remember tugging sweater sleeves down across my knuckles to cover the scrappy scars on my hands and wrists.

The self-mutilation started when I was eleven and continued sporadically through my teens. It would go away, and then come back when I had an intense period of depression; it was especially bad during my early twenties. After I met Jason, the compulsion stopped for about eight years, then returned when we moved to Cape Town during my early thirties.

Coming down painfully from four glorious months of summer mania once – I was about twenty-two or twenty-three – I felt isolated from the world. Back then, as soon as I felt the first tingling of mania, I'd throw out whichever boyfriend I was involved with. One Friday afternoon, feeling chaotic and bad, intimidated by the lack of reality in my life, I smashed a glass tumbler in the kitchen and started jabbing at the skin on my right hand, on the side of my palm. I cut and cut until finally I grew bored and bemused by the streams of blood. I wrapped my hand in an old T-shirt.

Later that night, outside the apartment, I bumped into a drunken neighbour who claimed to be a doctor and asked about my hand. She was also schizophrenic, gay and allegedly a devout Jew. She bandaged me up and we had a strange, drunken Shabbat dinner. I don't believe she really was a doctor, because I've still got the scar. It was a deep wound and should have had stitches. But she was cool, she was kind of gentle and, I suppose, she was too 'out there' herself to judge me.

The urge to self-mutilate vanished again as mysteriously as it had come, and for years there were no further incidents – a suicide attempt, yes, but no carving at my flesh.

Then, many years later, I was in hospital waiting for my husband Jason and to see the doctor. I'd been checked in the night before and had awoken at 6 a.m., bemused and horrified. The nursing staff couldn't give me any medication to calm me down until the doctor arrived. As ever, I desperately needed to be close to Jason and to be reassured by him.

I lay on a narrow bed in a sterile private ward. My breakfast, a plastic tray of inedible hospital food, lay next to me. There were no metal implements (never trust a psychiatric patient), so with deliberate calm I began to jab away at my right hand with a toothpick. My right side always takes the cuts, because I'm left-handed.

Jason used to have an absurd theory that you could murder a person with a toothpick. You can't. But you can dig, and you can dig quite far into the flesh before the toothpick mashes into split ends. And you can draw a reasonable amount of blood, creatively causing yet another whitening line of scar tissue.

I have no intimate or detailed recollection of these events. No dates, times, awareness or integrated reminiscences. My mind reveals only a fuzzy patchwork of other people's accounts of events, combined with the feathery white scars that map their way across my skin like rivers. So much took place when I wasn't quite there. It happened to another girl, who had nothing to do with me.

Sometimes, when I'm climbing out of the bath, I'll catch a glimpse of a jagged line etched somewhere on my body. These lines don't fade, despite the application of lotions and potions. I can't rub them away with vitamin E oil; they're tattooed on my skin, obstinate reminders of times I'd rather forget. When I see them I'm startled, taken aback by surprise. How did they get there? Amnesia is a gracious gift.

When I first tried to write about my self-mutilation, the narrative didn't come across in my own voice. Instead, I wrote in a detached, journalistic tone. That's not really surprising. These things happened to me as if in a dream, without conscious volition or decision. I no longer inhabited my own body. My frightened spirit had stepped outside of it in revulsion and now looked down from a giddy height. An astral traveller staring at a horror movie – scenes you can watch as entertainment because it is all happening to someone else, some-where else. No one should have to write about self-mutilation. It goes against the human condition.

Stepping out of my body and looking down on it has been a re-current theme in my life. Sometimes I did so in revulsion, sometimes in bliss. When I was younger and dancing regularly, there were days when hours of stretching and torturing my body would suddenly wake it to a life entirely its own. With the grace of a bird in free flight, possessed and impervious to my own exhaustion, my body would pirouette perfectly from one end of the studio to the other. My spirit hovered above me, gazing down in delight as a strange, mythical semblance of my physical self spun unhindered around the confines of the real world. It was a glorious sensation, but I feared that if I allowed this to happen too often and for too long, my spirit would become dislodged, even unhinged, from my body, and I would probably die.

Shortly after Valentine's Day, when I was thirty-three, I sat quivering in bed, staring at the strawberry bush Jason had given me as a romantic gift. It was now wilting pathetically, withering away. I couldn't bear the symbolic connection between the bush and me. The day had started with vigorous self-medication. A panic attack that refused to chill was abated with a combination of Xanor, Valium and Ativan (some pretty addictive tranquillisers).

The combination of drugs, along with stress, brought on a pounding headache, so I took a couple of analgesics. Self-medicating is a tricky business, particularly when orchestrated by the layman. My mood continued to lash out at me uninhibited, despite the medication, so I slid into a dangerous cocktail of drugs, downed recklessly: Xanor, Stopain, Imovane, Valium, Ativan, painkillers, Stilnox and Aropax.

That night Jason's producer came over with a video and a take-out dinner. Displaying a profound lack of insight – or a madness that rivalled mine – the film she brought was *Iris*, about the mental decline of the writer Iris Murdoch as her doting husband desperately cared for her. Although I didn't watch the movie, I'd read the reviews and knew what it was about. To me, the producer seemed to be implying that I was a manipulative female who was in control of what I was doing and willingly destroying my husband's life and art. I knew I wouldn't be able to watch the film with them, so I was left alone, which I perceived as being abandoned.

Every ten minutes, Jason would excuse himself from the film and run downstairs to confirm the beating of my broken heart. I was pretty out there, over-medicated, spinning and spinning out of my tree, spinning out of the entire forest. I convinced myself that the guest would come and check up on me, so I locked myself inside my cupboard. I threw every item of clothing I possessed onto the floor and chaotically began a frenzy of obsessive–compulsive folding, arranging everything into perfectly measured, colour-coded, categorised piles.

Upstairs, I could hear the tormenting chatter and laughter of an army. I needed Jason's comfort but couldn't risk calling him, couldn't risk having traffic with the talking, laughing enemy in my lounge, which seemed to have been invaded and was now an enemy camp. I was hiding out in the trenches of my dressing room.

Perhaps I was desperate for evidence of illness, a physical manifestation of what was happening to me, to externalise the chaos running rampant within, as though proof of pain would provide relief from it. I ventured nervously out of the cupboard and into the bedroom in search of a sharp object. Jason, no fool, had hidden everything except my Diet Coke can.

I took the tab you pull to open the can and began to cut away at my calf. When the blood started pouring too profusely for my squeamish nerves, I began to panic. Band-Aids, stored upstairs in the kitchen, were being held hostage in the enemy camp. One moment I was blotting and bandaging my leg with a precious cashmere sweater, and the next I resumed cutting, this time on the thigh of my other leg. Finally, my body exhausted, the cocktail of drugs kicked in, and I passed out onto a heap of neatly folded clothes on the floor.

When Jason saw the state I was in, he called my GP, who, unaware of all the medication I'd already taken, shot me up with Pethidine and Feldene. Half of this cocktail would normally sink a battleship. Yet, once awake, I remained overwrought and full of manic energy, tingling in wide-eyed desperation. One feature of psychosis is how impervious it is to medication. Nothing works. Ironically, nowadays I shy away from alcohol and tartrazine because of their toxicity.

Sunday morning, when my GP returned to tell Jason that he thought I'd be safest in hospital, I was pretty cut up. When Jason looked at me, he knew he was looking not at the face of his beloved wife, but into the face of madness. Swirling, swarming fear was trapped behind my eyes.

Once admitted to hospital, I continued to find inventive ways of cutting myself, as the ever-increasing dosage of medication continued to have little or no effect. Psychosis is nothing if not resilient.

I haven't cut myself for a long time. As I look out at the sunny begonias in the garden and relish the fragrance of freesias in a vase, I can't imagine myself doing such a tawdry, destructive thing again. It made no sense then, and it makes no sense now.

I flinch at the sight of my scars. I turn away from a movie screen to avoid the sight of blood in a film. I could barely bring myself to see *Iris* then, but when I finally watched that brilliant writer disintegrating into senile dementia, right from the opening moments to the closing credits I had a metallic taste in my mouth – the taste of shame and fear.

Scars heal – if not all the external ones, certainly the internal ones. Time, love, Mr Thomas Waits and fresh flowers are some of what it takes. Life conspires to heal me.

CHAPTER 10

A dirty, self-loathing sickness

Jason was thrown into the deep end right at the very beginning. When we met in September 1993, I was a tiny ball full of laughter. Then, one morning five months later, out of the blue, I woke up crying.

It may have been the recklessness of mania that threw a few cocktail dresses and stiletto heels into the back of Jason's car as we embarked on a road trip to Cape Town, but he just assumed the girl he'd fallen for didn't eat, sleep or stop talking. The crazy high continued for a couple of months, but, inevitably, by January it had softened. In February I started gaining weight and taking a horrifying cocktail of slimming drugs in an attempt to restore my energy levels and control my weight. To no avail. The ball was already rolling.

There was no stopping the cycle. The decline was inevitable. And on that March morning, when I woke crying for no reason, Jason was suddenly with a very different girl – one who constantly wept, slept like a newborn and couldn't ingest enough starch.

I'd also started vomiting. As a child my sisters used to tease me about my 'allergies, allergies', because I so often had my head in the toilet. I suppose my childhood vomiting was a nervous response, but we put it down to my 'sensitive constitution'. By my teenage years it seemed like all the girls did it on occasion. But when I started doing it regularly, it was in desperation, a manifestation of angst and terror. I was out of control.

When I was young, my father had once come home with enough bubble bath to fill the entire swimming pool. Naturally he ruined the filter, but for one glorious day our suburban pool was transformed into a giant scented bubble bath. That frothy day reminds me of mania, but the depression following a manic episode is like swimming in the pool after the filter had broken – everything is heavy and dark.

My eating patterns during those two phases were equally polarised. Mania was 'Sly Anna', who surreptitiously fed the dog her lunch under the table when no one was looking. Sadly, Sly Anna left along with the laughter of mania and was replaced by the weight of bulimia. If bulimia had a sound, it would be like the thud of the first spadeful of sand thrown onto a coffin in the ground. You can't see through bulimia – it has a kind of murky finality to it. Thud, it pulls you down with the weight of the ages.

Bulimia is grim, a dirty, self-loathing sickness. I'd sit alone on the kitchen floor with Capote, my long-haired miniature dachshund. We'd start at around midnight, an epic, disgusting binge that began with the baking of fudge and chocolate brownies. After the fudge, we'd move on to every bulimic's fallback favourite: toast. Eventually

I didn't bother to toast the bread or even defrost it properly – just swallowed hard on the frozen bits in the centre. Capote, always loyal and as greedy as me, would do a fine job of following suit, packing it in regardless of taste.

We failed to notice the healthy foods, the salads or fruit. They didn't have a role to play on this particular journey. I was so afraid and lonely, convinced that if I just kept eating I'd never have to leave the room, never again have to sit in auditions, as I had countless times since moving to Cape Town, waiting to say, 'Hi, I'm Rahla. I'm from Storm modelling agency. I'm 5.4 and I weigh 54 kilograms. Shoe size 5.' Never again have to be looked up and down by boys who were just as aware as I how precarious was my pedestal. A lipstick smudged, a kilogram gained, a blemish, a new girl in town – anything could topple me.

I gazed around the rapidly emptying kitchen, all the food pretty much flattened. My eyes rested longingly on the rat poison at the bottom of the broom cupboard – aah, to sleep, perchance to dream. To be rid of the pressure, the loneliness, the sense of debt, the emptiness. To be rid of the crippling hunger.

I was so full. So sick and tired, sleepy but unable to sleep. Capote looked up at me imploringly. One more lingering look at the box of rat poison and I headed for the toilet, toothbrush in hand, resigned to bringing it all up. To purge myself of the shame, the toxins and the guilt, rid myself of the fat. Maybe even momentarily be rid of myself.

I had a slimy gremlin living inside me. No matter how much food I gave him, he was never satiated. I'd stuff myself and stuff myself in a bid to drown him, but he'd just grow. Then I'd try to throw him out. Throw him up. But he stayed, fixed as he was inside me, inside my organs.

Thank God I eventually plucked up the courage to tell Jason about this nightly ritual. By that time, I'd quit my job and had pretty much quit life. Eating and vomiting four or five times a day isn't living. It isn't anything remotely related to life. Not unlike anorexia, bulimia leans closer towards death than it does to life.

Most young boys of twenty-four would have been repelled. Not Jason. He tackled the issue as he tackles everything: gently, kindly, but proactively. I'm an ostrich. God knows whether it's laziness or cowardice, but I'm not just a procrastinator, I'm a total denier. Jason is the opposite. As an idea enters his mind, he acts on it. He insisted we tell my parents. They had long suspected it. My family, as always, were compassionate.

The doctor gave a 'guarded prognosis'. In layman's terms, he wasn't prepared to guarantee that I'd live through it. My oesophagus had collapsed from the abuse, and I had the look of a bullfrog or a blowfish because of the swollen glands around my throat. My hands were calloused and I vomited blood. Later in life I'd lose a lot of my teeth, as the acids produced by the stomach during excessive vomiting cause tooth decay. My hair had thinned and my skin was chalky. I felt cumbersome in my body and cumbersome in the world. When I moved at all, I kind of lugged about.

I thought that in acknowledging the problem I'd done my share of the hard work. Now the professionals would step in and make it better. But acknowledging it is only step one. Then you must begin to live and work with the professionals and the illness.

Bulimia is like being in a crowded shopping mall, with a heavy-metal band playing full blast and everything speeded up. I don't believe that the sufferer can go it alone. Stuck in the trenches, soldiers don't usually stand up, rip off their uniforms, throw cake at one another and make white flags out of their underpants as the English and the Germans miraculously did in December 1914. No, they shit themselves. They say ten Hail Marys and shoot. Bulimia is fighting on the battlefield. It's a daily battle. Every day the victim empowers new enemies, and then has to fight them off in order to survive.

Often, in misguided attempts to make me feel better, people would say things like, 'You alone have the power to make yourself better.' That frightened me more than anything else. I had been waging war in solitude for months. If I could have done it alone, I sure as hell would have kept the battle to myself.

Eating disorders, drug addiction and alcoholism – maybe they're all different responses to the same stuff, that which disempowers a person. When people cry for help, they need help. Only later, when their health is improved and the wolf is at bay, can they get in touch with their inner strength.

I don't believe any of us should ever have to get better from anything on our own. As a species, we support one another. That's part of the joy of humanity. Ultimately, yes, I know all that stuff about coming into this world alone and going out of this world alone and you go to bed alone at night and blah, blah, blah. But sometimes people come and tuck you in, and that's cool.

Two years before my confession to Jason, the sky had embraced my light body as the ground elevated me. I'd been Icarus in free flight. It had started with a diet. Dieting was effortless. In fact, it wasn't long before eating seemed like rather a silly thing to do, a waste of precious time. The ingestion of food became disgusting, stupid.

As food went out the door, so, too, did sleep. I'd be up all night baking – ironically – dancing in the kitchen, listening to Radio Metro, the late, late show. I was wired to the moon. I felt immortal, unencumbered by mundane needs like nutrition or rest. I was divine. I felt more like me than I'd ever felt. It seemed that my body had been inhabited by another girl my whole life.

My pants were falling off my delicate frame. I secured them with a piece of rope, like a sailor. I loved the feeling of being thin. My brain was like a sharpened blade; I could cut through to the core of things. Things that other people couldn't fathom were clear and simple to me. I was concise, with millions of ideas whooshing constantly through my fertile mind. I didn't filter any of them. I just spewed them out in a crazy dance of frenetic chaos. No one could tie me down. I flew. I was so close to the sun that its rays energised me, making me more exuberantly alive.

But of course all was not really well. One night, I collapsed from malnourishment. The following day I landed up with Dr X, a psychiatrist. It was a Monday afternoon. The air smelt of a Highveld storm and rain marbled the view of the doctor's garden I could see through the window. I was safe, warm and dry. It had been so long since I had eaten that my mouth was parched.

Soothing classical music was playing. Fresh jasmine tumbled out of a terracotta vase onto the table. I soon blotted out its lingering scent with the foul smell of cigarettes. I could taste my putrid breath. Bad breath from smoking and not eating.

The doctor listened to my stories. He was kind and accessible, appeared not to judge. He said I had anorexia. That was cool. I had friends who'd had it. I thought it was a sign of a strong will; rather admirable, really. I was happy and satisfied with what I considered a glamorous diagnosis. I think I thought I couldn't also be fat if I had anorexia.

So it wasn't haphazard, this starvation. It had a name: anorexia. Everyone else had suspected anorexia for some time. The doctor was gentle, as though I may find the news shocking.

Now, two years on, after all my bingeing and purging, my dirty midnight secret, my crashing and confessing to Jason, I was back at another doctor. Another diagnosis. There were no photos, no ornaments and certainly no flowers here. Dr Y was kind. They were always kind. We talked and talked, or at least I talked and he nodded vigorously in agreement. He explained me to me. Youngest of five children, a lifetime of dancing, the odd stint in front of a camera – eating disorders, it seemed, were almost inevitable. I didn't care; I just wanted to feel the unbearable lightness of being, I wanted to go back to being manic, even though I didn't yet know what 'mania' was or of the dangers it held.

Dr Y was keen on eating disorders. He was knowledgeable about dysfunctions surrounding women and food. When he diagnosed me as bulimic, Princess Di had it too, so bulimia was kind of all the rage. Society seems to go through 'it' psychiatric phases. I'm not sure if it's because pharmaceutical companies come up with new drugs or because celebrities 'come out' with their crazies. What I do know is that until I was correctly diagnosed as bipolar, I was a serial psychiatric patient.

Medicating me was simple. The 'it' diagnosis of bulimia came with the 'it' drug. Princess Di had come out in favour of Prozac. In high doses it helped to curb binge-eating. Later, much later, I was to find out that in high doses it also tripped the light fantastic into mania. Whoopie.

Dr Y referred me to a dietician. I arrived forty minutes late, but felt soothed by the music, the cool breeze, the fresh roses. She was pretty and she spoke gently.

'When you have an eating disorder, it's all darkness, and people say that there's a light at the end of the tunnel, but for you it's only darkness. There are flashlights, little torches you can hold, people who will guide you through the tunnel, giving you enough light to put one foot in front of the other. That's all you can do. Put one foot in front of the other, take one step at a time, one day at a time.'

For the first time in months I felt a sense of hope, of safety and of an imminent journey.

Zhan, the dietician, came into my life like an angel. She taught me how to eat, one mouthful at a time. She reminded me how to chew and swallow. It was terrifying. From anorexia to bulimia, my relationship with food was turbulent both physically and emotionally. I couldn't remember when last I'd felt genuine hunger and responded by eating. I approached food as a child reacts to an abusive parent.

Zhan's slow pace was appropriate for me. She worked instinctively, healing and teaching, healing and teaching. She drew charts and pictures. She treated me like a child. On many levels, that's what eating disorders do. They reduce you to the helplessness of a child.

I started to make my environment calmer. One day I saw an advertisement in the paper for a nursery school teacher in a small town called Rustenburg. I phoned the headmistress. She liked my CV, so I caught a bus to Rustenburg and fell in love. The school had an aviary at its entrance. The children were all barefoot. They had grubby clothes and clean, shiny faces.

The logistics didn't enter my mind. I didn't know how to drive. I didn't know where I would live. I was by no means cured. Jason and I had been together for about one-and-a-half years. He and his family supported me. My family were nervous. But I went and it was the best thing I could have done.

My two years in Rustenburg were of the happiest in my life. I felt sheltered and loved. My class was called the Rabbits. My classroom was decorated in pink and green. Jason's stepmother lovingly made curtains and cushions with fabric depicting bunnies playing in a field of pink flowers. Just as my relationship with Jason provided a safe environment, so did the school, the teachers, the

parents and the children. The children were unspoilt, unsophisti-
cated and very loving. Jason wrote school plays and I directed them.
Living in a small town worked well for me.

During my years in Rustenburg, I finally learnt to drive. My eating normalised. My confidence was boosted. I wrote cars off with
alarming regularity, but I managed not to injure anyone. I saved (for
the first time in my life) enough money to put down a deposit and
buy myself a new car. I wrote it off after a week. But the act of
buying it was swell.

Life wasn't *all* light and breezy. There were periods of loneliness
and despair. But generally my life was toned down; so quiet that it
accommodated my feelings and successfully kept most emotional
turbulence at bay.

Towards the end of the second year, I was ready to approach
reality again, and we moved back to Johannesburg. Jason and I
found a little house with roses in the garden. We went on holiday
to the Seychelles. I panicked that Jason would never marry me. He
panicked that he would. In May, I gave him an ultimatum. In June,
he gave me a ring. We moved into a fancier, bigger house with all
sorts of flowers in the rambling, frolicking garden.

Then my mood wobbled. I went into denial. I discovered Ayurveda. I did extensive rebirthing and breathing work. I was told that
because I was always convinced I'd been an unplanned baby, I'd
never felt welcome in the world and, as a result, I was breeched at
birth. I had to be hypnotised to relive the trauma of being born.
I relived it all in my bathtub. My mood went into free fall, down,
down, down, but not to where the iguanas play. I remained in
denial. I was studying to become an Ayurvedic practitioner, but this
didn't protect me. Nothing, it seemed, could protect me. My mood
crashed to the solitude of the bottom.

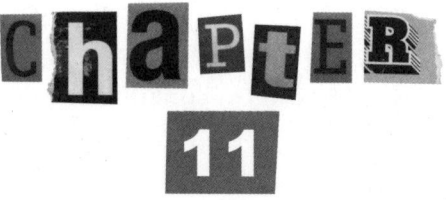

CHAPTER 11

My heart belongs to Daddy

On Sunday mornings we all used to make a dash for my parents' bedroom. Each child got a chance to sit on Daddy's knees; he'd hold our little hands like reins. The sun shone in through the window, hazy with minute particles of dust.

Daddy would sing, 'She's got rings on her fingers, bells on her toes, elephants to ride upon, my little Irish rose.' It never occurred to me to wonder who the Irish rose was or why she needed an elephant to ride upon, because the smell of jasmine, the love and laughter twinkling in the sparkly make-believe eyes that held the reflection of my laughing morning face, made me an enchanted princess in an enchanted kingdom. And it was enough.

One perfect spring morning years later, Gigi phoned. 'Rahls, I've got bad news. It's Daddy. He's died.'

I cannot describe the absolute shock of my father's death. Nothing in life prepares us for the mortality of our parents. From early childhood we're taught to revere them, to defer to them on every dilemma. In adolescence we're conditioned to rebel against them. But even the act of rebellion is an act of respect. They're important enough to rebel against. Nothing in our society teaches us that they will die, that they won't always be around to debate with and love and have revolving around us unconditionally. My father was so much larger than life that he seemed to transcend the laws of nature. He'd been sick so many times before, but this time it was flu, and his body simply stopped fighting.

Jason and I had just got engaged. My last grand memory is of the speech Daddy made at our engagement party, when he spoke about Jason being a Renaissance man. Now he was gone, so suddenly, so suddenly.

That night all of us congregated around the familiar old Georgian dining table. All except for David, who had yet to arrive on an aeroplane from Israel. I was still wearing the emerald-green dress I'd worn to take my exam to be an Ayurvedic practitioner. It occurred to me that Daddy would never see the dress or watch me practising Ayurveda. He wouldn't walk me down the aisle or carry my baby or make Livicky laugh again. She wouldn't laugh; no, she wouldn't laugh again.

We ate food that kind friends and neighbours had brought for us. After a death, there's suddenly so much food, as though eating will bring the loved one back. All too suddenly we were basking in the crazy legacy he'd left, a legacy of love. He didn't make money and he didn't make sense, but he made magic.

That Friday night around the table, a summation of all the Friday-night dinners of our lives, we all made perfect sense of it. We dealt with his death the way he had taught us to live: by laughing and loving and eating and talking nonsense and having great, glorious memories of the world he had brought us all into. 'Child, hold my hand that I may walk in the light of your faith in me.' And so we walked and lived and danced in the divine light that Daddy had carried around in his relenting heart.

There was always excitement and a sense of occasion surrounding Daddy. Children were drawn to him; he was terribly funny and not entirely predictable. Daddy ran his practice in a surgery upstairs, and sometimes he would come down from work at 10 p.m. and take us all in our pyjamas and slippers to Chinatown to celebrate his brilliant matric results – achieved thirty years previously. He sang. And he made us all laugh. He adored my mother. He insisted that we, the siblings, should never fight. Thank God we don't.

I always valued my family and I rather enjoyed being Jewish. I love the traditions. I love the emphasis on family values and I love to light candles on a Friday night to bless the new week. After my father's death, my family and my religion made the process of mourning bearable. The Jewish way of mourning is called sitting *shiva*. Every night for seven nights people came to the house to say prayers with the family. The rituals carried us through, picking us up and guiding us, step by step, through each emotion.

I was amazed at the incredible amount of love that poured forth. All my father ever held dear in the world was love – and that was his legacy. He had had a successful life, because he had realised his dream. People loved him; people around him loved one another. He might have left a financial mess, but all the people in his life were bundled up in love. Daddy neither cared for nor understood money. He was a people person. People filled our house at prayers for Daddy, and the overflow of the crowd stood in the garden.

We, the Fensters, cried a lot, but I think we laughed even more.

I love my family. As a tribe, I think we are a marvel. I think we are the funniest, cleverest, happiest, craziest family in God's entire green universe.

Daddy enabled our childlike faith in the world as a candy-coated journey, the belief that people are intrinsically good and want to help. Seeing the world through rose-tinted lenses was not only sensible, but the *only* way to look at life. Happy endings are the only logical conclusions, and never-never land exists wherever you lay your head.

Once, Livicky was abroad looking after her mother. We were left in the care of the domestic worker, Melita, and Daddy. We ate takeaways from Bimbos and ice cream from Milky Lane. Pnina got everybody to enter the *Sunday Times* colouring-in competition. A couple of days later we were playing in the garden when a twinkling strand of candy hanging out of the postbox caught David's eye. On closer inspection it was discovered that the postbox was literally overflowing with sweets. Daddy explained that it was our prize for winning the colouring-in competition. Many years later, as we sat around the table at *Shabbat*, Gigi said, 'Daddy, we didn't really win the *Sunday Times* colouring-in competition, did we?' But it didn't matter, because all our lives we were the winners in the golden glow of Daddy's light.

Of course there were flashes of twilight and uncertainty in my childhood. Daddy was expansive and funny, but his temper surprises me even now, in recollection, because it seemed to have had nothing to do with his naturally compassionate, gentle personality.

A common trait among doctors is an inclination to self-medicate, and he was not beyond it. Sometimes after nights of relentless insomnia he'd knock himself out with a sleeping pill for at least a day. Then appointments would be cancelled and the world would shut down. I don't recall the household falling silent, but we knew something was wrong with Daddy. He'd been working too hard, worrying too much, wasn't well physically. Livicky knew what to do with him. We didn't. Sometimes even she didn't.

Then he'd wake up and we'd hear Livicky's laughter resounding through the house, the neighbourhood and even − or so it seemed − the world. Daddy would bundle us up in our pyjamas and take us to Café Wien to eat slices of Black Forest cake.

When I was in high school, I got a casual job waitressing on Saturday mornings. Until then, Saturday mornings had been reserved for Daddy and me to spend time together while my mother taught. One morning, he came into the restaurant and ordered a black filter coffee. When I brought him the bill, he said, 'How much do they pay you in this dive? What about I double it and we split to the movies?' Even to me, his daughter, his charm was irresistible and his logic irrefutable. So he paid the bill and we bolted.

On Sunday afternoons, when the streets of Johannesburg's suburbs were deserted, we'd drive home from his ward rounds at the clinics and he'd play the soundtrack of *A Chorus Line* on the car stereo. We'd go dancing in his navy-blue Peugeot, swerving left to right along the broad streets framed by jacaranda trees. With a carpet of purple blossoms popping under the wheels, he'd swerve the car gracefully in time to the lyrics, 'One thrilling combination ...'

He was famous for being fun. It was only after his death, as I began to examine my own mood swings, my own expansive, impulsive behaviour, that I recognised the similarities in our patterns.

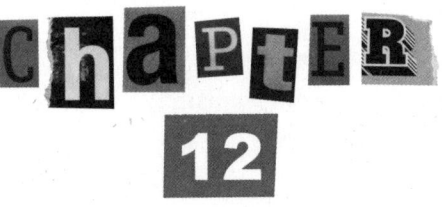

CHAPTER 12

Backwards into the darkness

November is a tricky month. It's the month of my birthday, and I'm an old-fashioned birthday girl. I love the passing of the years that are marked with kitsch candled cakes, taffeta-ribboned packets and long-distance phone calls. The sky is always so bright and full of summer promise in November. But the November sun often also brings with it the harsh rays of warning, the tap, tap, tapping away at my psyche, the feeling of dis-ease, discomfort nagging at my soul. All the excitement has a sort of dark lining; it's all kind of touch and go.

On one particular November Friday, it was not so much touch as it was go, go, go … vroom, vroom, vroom. I woke, went to gym and then did a million unnecessary, frenetic things. If anything was wrong with me, it was being too 'up'. I thought I was possibly a bit manic. At the time I was going through a liquorice phase – Panda liquorice with its picture of a cute panda – stockpiling black-and-yellow boxes of the stuff.

I was hanging beads and eating liquorice when Jason said good-bye, off to do some work. A bit nervous, I dropped the beads and followed him, Panda in hand, to say goodbye. As he got into the car, I started to cry. I tried to explain: What would I do when my Panda was finished? No, I didn't just want to go to the shops and buy a new box, because I loved that particular box. Then I was crying inconsolably for the inevitable loss of my Panda liquorice. Within an hour I was hysterical, truly off my trolley.

Psychiatrists have lives independent of their patients, so they're not always contactable on a Friday night. My Cape Town psychiatrist was out of town, but we got hold of the Happy Potter doctor in Johannesburg. He said, 'Go to hospital and try to get some food into yourself while you're there.'

Take a psychotic person to a regular hospital and nobody really wants to take responsibility. My father used to say that hospitals aren't too keen to give beds to psychiatric patients because hospitals are run like hotels. In any hotel, the bar brings in the money. With hospitals, the bar is the operating theatre. So, unless you're having electroconvulsive treatment or you need an anaesthetist, you're essentially just wasting precious bed space. But Jason, long-suffering Jason, managed to get me, still clutching my liquorice, across town and admitted to hospital. So much of this is just a blur. I have a fabulous way of forgetting. Daddy used to say, 'You don't always need a good memory; sometimes you need a good forgettory!'

I'm a gifted amnesiac. I remember in minute detail every birthday and anniversary celebration. I remember childhood happenings and everything to do with my friends' lives. But the recollections I have of depressive episodes are fractured. Always, I recall the feeling of people's care and support. I remember trying to pass the pain of time by watching outdated but funny movies like the Marx Brothers and trying to keep my anxiety focused on just one thing: my incessant beading – long strands of crystals and pink shimmering baubles. I would concentrate intently on stringing one bead after another.

I remember the smell of fresh roses, but not the putrid decay of my despair. The details of getting into a hospital bed draw a blank. How did my clothes get there? Did Jason pack them with me, or did he bring them the next day? How did he know what to pack? What did he do with my dogs? What did he tell the neighbours? I have no idea.

Mornings that I thought were the preceding day were in fact the following evening. Days became weeks, which are lost. In this way I've misplaced years of my life, and maybe it's just as well. When you enter a depressive episode you enter the twilight zone, and amnesia is a blessing, a God-given tool of survival.

I'm sure many psychologists would say that I'm in a state of denial and that I should face what has happened. But I'm grateful for what I can forget. If the darkness is visible, cool, I'll look it in the eye. But if it vanishes into nowhere, well, that's also fine, because I want to live in this world, not in the melancholy nothingness of illness. To write about it, though, I need to try to step backwards, into the darkness.

Saturday morning I woke in a strange hospital bed, alone, afraid, no Jason, no doctor, just despair and an empty breakfast tray with a toothpick staring at me. I think people get suicidal in hospital because it is last-resort territory – the end of the road. It's what you get when all else fails. There's this myth that if you go to hospital, all those doctors and nurses in their chirpily starched outfits are going to take control. The nurses, so smart and contained, their shoes so shiny, the corridors of their wards so polished that they can see their reflected faces. They'll take the troubling malady away, but if they can't, oh God, if *they* can't make you better, who can?

The next day, three friends came with Jason to visit me. One brought long-stemmed roses, a shiny gold box of Lindt chocolates and a huge bag of popcorn. That I remember. Then it's a blur – days of doctors trying to medicate my mood while friends tried to make me smile. Until the psychiatrist recommended moving me from the psychiatric ward in the regular hospital to a special psychiatric clinic, where the doctors and nurses were trained to attend to me 24/7.

There was something awful about that place. In the normal hospital, I could pretend I was there for 'other' reasons. Reasons 'other' than being insane. But that place – it was *One Flew Over the Cuckoo's Nest*, it was *Girl, Interrupted*.

I remember the smell: musty, chlorinated, with whiffs of cheap air-freshener. The registration form upset me, because I had to promise that I'd never communicate with any of the other patients after I checked out. I didn't even want to communicate with them inside, they all looked so weird. There was a communal bathroom. The curtains in the room were a shade of vomit brown. A girl came and touched my hair, saying, '*Is dit die nuwe meisie?*' (Is this the new girl?) All this I remember. I can touch my fear.

When Jason left, I wanted to die. I didn't want to kill myself; I simply wanted to be dead. Did I make it through a full night in that place? I'm not sure. By the following day, however, I was out of the psychiatric clinic and back in the regular hospital, with its regular nurses. The psychiatrist had had the good sense to test my thyroid – thyroid problems and mood disorders apparently are best friends. If anything, my thyroid at that stage indicated overactivity. I was keen as mustard on the diagnosis, knowing that an overactive thyroid made you skinny. The doctor suspected that the thyroid might change direction. But things got better and my mood improved day by day, until I was discharged.

Livicky came to Cape Town to be with me. Psychiatrists may be unavailable when you need them the most, but my mother is always available. Realities of life, work responsibilities – none of it exists. When I need her, she's there.

Free of the hospital again, I had a fabulous birthday, a glorious social summer. I felt cool. But the decline was insidious.

As so often happens, my mood was triggered by weight gain. I felt my jeans getting snug, looked in the mirror and thought my face looked fat. Stood on the scale and counted the extra God-forbidden numbers. Then I decided not to go to the beach because I couldn't face being in a bikini. I became less and less motivated, lazier and lazier. One by one, activities were cancelled out of my life. One day I was sick and missed a session with my trainer. She was nasty about it, and Gigi said, 'I refuse to let you be upset by someone with a brain the size of a pea.'

But it wasn't just gym. Everything became more of an effort. I was flat but not quite depressed. I ascribed it to the change in medication. After all the fuss of November's episode, I refused to entertain the idea that anything else could be wrong. For days I just slept. Slept and ate. By January, I started to get concerned. I under-went a series of tests. I had a thyroid virus: Hashimoto's thyroiditis, an autoimmune condition. For some unknown reason, the body fails to recognise the thyroid as its own organ and treats it like an invader. The misguided immune system then bombards the gland until the virus ensues. The condition is triggered by stress.

I always feel guilty when I'm depressed, particularly in hospital. It feels like I'm copping out of life. Everybody else is working and functioning in the world while I'm catatonic, crying, needing to be taken care of. But whereas a week in a hydro is relaxing, a week in a depression leaves you drained and exhausted. The misconception is that a person who has stepped out of the stresses of day-to-day life has removed herself from stress. In fact, she has stepped into the most stressful chaos imaginable: chaos that comes without respite, relentless chaos because it's not caused by the screeching of car breaks or the moaning of bosses; it comes from inside, it comes from the place that doesn't end at the end of the day.

I'm appalled at how many educated, intelligent people envy me my condition. How often they've said, 'God, you're so lucky! I wish I could take a few days' timeout.' Make no mistake – this is not a timeout. This is war. This is fighting a merciless battle amidst despair and nothingness. But there's no blood, no physical evidence of injury.

We live in such a physical, tangible world in which everything has been scientifically proven. We want hard evidence, or we can't believe. Sometimes I think that's why I cut myself, to create a physical manifestation of pain so that I can wipe away the blood and apply a plaster.

If there's nothing broken or bloodied, then what's wrong? Often I admonish myself, 'There's nothing wrong. Snap out of it. You're just feeling sorry for yourself.' But saying those things only makes it a longer, harder journey. Self-love is the biggest *schlep*, the hardest part of all.

My body was feeling the knocks, because by January it was in rebellion. The thyroid virus was the body fighting itself. The doctor explained that there was nothing we could do. We just had to wait it out. I waited. I lay around waiting, me with my obscure sickness. I can never just get flu. No, it has to be some weird, off-the-wall sickness with a strange name.

My hair started falling out. I put on nine kilos. I was too exhausted to leave the house and, if I did, I had panic attacks. I got more and more depressed. By February I had the crying germ, another full-blown depression.

My GP came to the house to administer injections for the migraines and the anxiety, but my desolation remained impervious to help. Eventually he recommended hospital again as the best solution. This trip back to the hospital is a blur.

The psychiatrist tried and tried. Eventually he suggested ECT (electroconvulsive treatment, or 'shock treatment', as it is sensationally named). We've probably all seen Janet Frame's *Angel at my Table*, *One Flew over the Cuckoo's Nest* or *The Bell Jar*. For some reason, ECT is a very cinematic procedure. The camera loves the convulsions of the body, much as it loved Marilyn Monroe's curves. I think it's a procedure that's been given a pretty bad rap. The way it's depicted is always so archaic. Sure, it's horrific, but, gee whiz, make no mistake, so is depression.

I used to have an aversion to the idea of ECT, but I began to read more about it and over the years my feelings towards it softened. I spoke to people who swore that it had saved their lives, that it was the only catalyst out of despair. I used to suspect that it penetrated and shocked the patient's spirit with lasting repercussions, but the sadness I'd known had also penetrated the very core of my spirit and shocked it indelibly.

My Cape Town psychiatrist was at a loss; nothing he did seemed to make any difference. A week and a half had passed and I hadn't improved. Livicky and my sister started saying that I should go back to the Happy Potter doctor in Johannesburg. I said that there was no way I could fly in that state. The Happy Potter doctor phoned Livicky. 'Rahla is terribly sick. She must come here immediately.'

A good friend came and talked me through it. Another packed my bags, while a helpful neighbour booked the ticket, drove me to the airport and physically put me on the plane. Jason packed up my hospital room. Gigi and her kids were at the airport in Johannesburg, waiting for me, and Livicky was at the clinic. I was carried through the chaos by love.

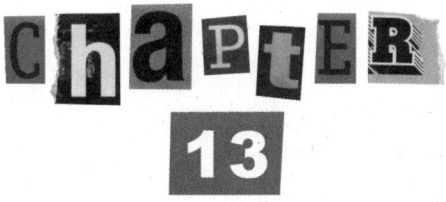

CHAPTER 13

More Happy Potter

One morning a couple of weeks later, after I'd waded through rivers of pain and sadness, the Happy Potter doctor smiled his familiar warm greeting. 'You've got a good smile,' he said.

I scanned the tubs of pencils for any new stationery to fiddle with, trying not to look nervous. 'Oh, how do you judge the behaviour of a person's smile?'

'That's a healthy smile,' he said.

I thought, 'Oh, that's rich. You still smile like a Teletubby,' but put on a deadpan face and asked, 'What are the criteria for a healthy smile?'

He looked at me with empathetic eyes, behind which I knew

an unseen universe was quietly going on. He discreetly made some notes in his weird psychiatric code.

'It's spontaneous, not too over the top, not too up, sincerely happy and relaxed. Not contrived and forced. It's just right. No anxiety. A happy, healthy smile.'

'Yes, well, that's hunky-dory, but I'm also scatterbrained, lacking in direction and terribly lazy.'

'Does that matter? You have your health.'

Not appreciating the sentiment, I leant over and grabbed a pen shaped like a long Prozac pill. 'Well, it doesn't seem right. I just lie at the pool all day ordering cappuccinos. It's ridiculously indulgent.'

He laughed. 'Nice work if you can get it, Rahla. You're recovering from a long period of seriously debilitating depression, and it might be a little while before you conquer the moon.'

Until that moment I'd pretty much forgotten just how bad I'd been feeling a week or so before. 'It's not that I'm ungrateful. I love that my mood is good. I appreciate that I've stopped crying. But my brain, she's all over the show!'

'Are you feeling a bit blonde about the brain? Well, that could be a few things. It could be the Topamax, an anti-epileptic that has the miraculous side effect of working as a mood stabiliser. Or it could be the Luvox, an antidepressant with a soporific effect.

'And then it could also be the after-effects of depression. When you're depressed, your brain cells temporarily stop regenerating,' he said.

'I don't care,' I said, chewing unconsciously on the Prozac pen, 'it's dull. Anyway, I blame the Luvox. I'm so lethargic.'

'Maybe next week we can look at decreasing the nightly Luvox and replacing it with twenty-five milligrams of extra Wellbutrin.'

Trying not to make it obvious how keen I was on that idea, as Wellbutrin makes me a bit up and takes the edge off my appetite, I said, 'That could work.'

He laughed. 'Yes, I thought you might like that idea. Wellbutrin is a skinny drug. Yesterday I gave a woman of ninety-two a prescription and she asked me if the medication would make her fat. You women are all mad. The god of pharmacology doesn't appreciate the emaciated female form!'

Shit, I thought, he'd seen through me now. 'I just want enough energy to visit my husband on set,' I told him, 'and no, I wouldn't mind fitting into my jeans and having my own functioning brain, pharmacologically maintained or otherwise.'

'Your problem is that your natural state is higher than the rest of ours. You're chirpy. It's a kind of ongoing soft mania.'

I replaced the Prozac pen and picked up the broken Montblanc of my early consultations. It still didn't work, which I found oddly comforting, because neither did I. Although I'd come a long way, the whole business was confusing. It took truckloads of psychotropic drugs to get me out of my depression and truckloads of psychotropic drugs to get me back to my own naturally, slightly manic – not *too* manic – state. Ordinary girl, I am an ordinary girl.

The doctor interrupted my reverie. 'The film industry isn't at all bipolar friendly, you know. Maybe 70 per cent of the people in it are bipolar, but they're what we call 'toxicity level' bipolars. Fake bipolars. A few months cleaned up and out of the industry, and if they haven't done indelible damage, they'd be absolutely fine.'

'Oh. And where does all of that leave me?' I found the notion of people willingly creating the mayhem I have to conquer in order to live entirely annoying.

'You should be writing it all down. Look at Stephen King. He only writes five hours a day and he makes a modest living.'

I replaced the pens and gave an amused smile. 'Ja, ja, thanks for the career advice, can I have the new script?'

'Let's wait and see your smile next week.'

As I left, the voice-over in my head said, 'Writing is all fine and well, but what are you writing towards? It doesn't matter, just write yourself out of it, and write yourself out of the funk, out from the inertia, away from the pink palace, down the yellow brick road and home to never-never land. Rahla, go home and write.'

As it turned out, the Happy Potter doctor had decided to use other treatments instead of ECT, so that option is still out there, waiting for a very rainy day. He had a theory: 'In psychiatry, when in doubt, think.' He had taken one look at me that first evening, at my sad eyes, and said he was going away to think. The next morning he'd thrown away the tablets for migraines and the tablets for panic attacks. The morning after that he'd cut down the dosage of one of the mood stabilisers. And gradually he'd started to clean me out.

Eventually, he announced his intention to detox me completely. I'm a born quitter – I've quit tobacco, drugs, alcohol, red meat, chicken, sugar, shopping and even mania! I love quitting, so I embraced the quitting of psychiatric medication with huge enthusiasm. At times I crave a purity of form; I hanker after a non-toxic, healthy lifestyle. Often I thought the only contradiction was the fourteen or so pills I took a day. Quitting them was a joy.

A full-blown depressive episode totally takes it out of you. Each episode has its own special reason for being the worst, most shattering experience of your life. But now that this particular episode was behind me, I convinced myself that I was cured, even though I had no foundation for my theory. It was clearly explained to me: you're experiencing a honeymoon period, a 'window period' in the illness. After a very bad episode, sometimes there's a respite in the illness, a stage where the patient is naturally normal and stable, but not cured.

For the first time, there was a new goal in sight. The Happy Potter doctor told me that he thought this was my chance for the baby I had wanted so desperately for so many years. He explained that the window period would allow time for me to fall pregnant. If we could hold off any psychiatric mishaps until my first trimester was completed, then everything would be fine. Typically, I didn't doubt that everything would go perfectly according to plan. Motherhood felt right. My only concern was that baby names wouldn't be ready on time.

Jason had been terrified of having a baby, but when I told him what the doctor had said, he didn't hesitate.

Now may be the time to mention that very few marriages sustain mental illness. Very little mental illness can sustain marriage. Invariably they are mutually exclusive.

A friend of mine threw her husband and his belongings out of the house during a manic episode. Mania gives a person an enormous supply of confidence and energy. You're so driven and proactive, it feels as if you can take on the entire world. My friend's manic cycle lasted long enough for her to sleep with her husband's best friend and get the divorce proceedings started. By the time she crashed back down to reality, it was too late. She'd wrapped it all up: years of marriage, homemaking and child-rearing. The marriage was *Oise Yom Tov*. Over, finished, a casualty of mania.

Holding a relationship together through the ups is one thing, but depression really tests romantic love. During tough episodes I've barely existed as a human being, bubble-wrapped in gloom, crying, cutting at my flesh, an inexplicable misery to everyone, while Jason has continued to function in the world, keep the house going, earn a living, pay the bills and make excuses to everyone for my bizarre retreat. Depressed people emanate a dark energy that's draining and exhausting.

Oddly, when I first come out of a depression, I assume everything is completely cool. In reality, that re-emergence and the re-establishment of normal relations is a huge adaptation, almost like getting reacquainted with my partner and learning to trust one another all over again.

That time, the time of my 'honeymoon period', I left the Happy Potter doctor in Johannesburg and flew back to Cape Town, but Jason wasn't at the airport to meet me. I didn't think he might be caught in peak-hour traffic; I simply assumed he didn't want me home at all. But he did want me and he did get through the traffic. He even got through my resentment and anxiety at not being collected on time.

None of it was easy. The doctor had told Jason, 'Okay, this is the time. You now have approximately three months to make a baby, and if she doesn't get pregnant in these three months, well, it's now or probably never.' It was no small amount of pressure for a man. Jason had just finished shooting a film and wasn't feeling financially secure. I can't imagine he was feeling too confident about his wife as a mother, either.

We tried doing the 'getting to know you routine' in Cape Town. After a couple of days we threw the dogs in the back of the car and drove to Plettenberg Bay. We're happy when we're together. It's the simplest recipe for a successful life. We love each other, relish each other's company. We were in a cocoon of love, having loads of sex in the required positions. Baby-making was the order of the day.

But I didn't fall pregnant. Perhaps we should have gone straight to a fertility clinic, but I didn't want to become neurotic and worry too much about not conceiving. I rationalised that possibly my medication had been working overtime as a contraceptive for the previous six years. But I believed it was going to happen. I imagined my fantasy daughter Tallulah packing her *petlach* in heaven. I was so steadfast, so confident. I was so sure that I was never again going to take another psychiatric drug, because I was cured. Miraculously, marvellously cured.

The Happy Potter doctor had explained carefully about the window period, but I didn't believe it, not a word. For roughly five months I was clean, clean, clean. I noticed a difference in my brain. On medication I'd always thought through a bit of a fog, a haze. Off it, my brain was clear. Cerebrally, it was bliss. I didn't constantly misplace my car in parking lots and I remembered people's names. My skin had a healthy glow and there were no bags under my eyes.

But I was on edge. I knew my mood was unprotected. When I opened my eyes in the morning it was like looking out at the view from the edge of a fifty-storey building. I happily conducted my days from the edge of that building, but for five months I knew that my feet weren't on the ground emotionally.

Worse, I continued to get fat and remained stubbornly un-pregnant. Eventually, in desperation, I went to a fertility clinic in Johannesburg. Jason was in pre-production for a feature film, so I felt rather alone. A series of tests showed that falling pregnant wasn't going to happen easily. We had things to fix. I felt the fragile thread of my mood slipping further and further away. I don't just wake up one morning in a state of semi-consciousness and want to die. It creeps up on me. There are warnings, sinister signs.

It's like when you leave a dish in the oven for too long and you can smell it burning, but you think that when you retrieve it, it'll be okay, you can just scrape off the edges. But it's a foregone conclusion; it's out of your hands. I try. I burn incense, I buy flowers, I exercise, I go to the movies, but I can smell the burning of brain cells and I'm just a small, silly, insignificant girl thing trying to fight off Alexander the Great's armies with cosmetics.

I thought, 'We've got this small chance of getting naturally pregnant; it's going to be fine.' But slowly, with each day that I visited the fertility clinic, with each procedure and each doctor I tried to smile at, the reality of being in a window period and not in a miraculous cure began to hit home. The window was getting smaller and darker.

We met with two experts in a calm, beige office. With great compassion they told us that Jason and I would never have children. The scientific facts fell out of their mouths with such authority and ease. Great care they showed, but the truth was definitive. They gave us options – adoption and surrogacy – and then sent us away, Jason in his car to a studio, me in mine to a hotel room. I was shattered. Any pretence of holding it together fell apart.

My body was so completely cleaned out, I thought that it would be like a dry sponge and absorb the new drugs immediately. But I found out that mood stabilisers don't work like Ecstasy. It takes two to six weeks for the medication to kick in. Two weeks of sitting in a hotel room contemplating my barren womb.

Maybe God had a different plan for me, one that didn't involve my lifelong ambition for motherhood. And who was I to question the Divine? There were so many other considerations: movies to be made, houses to be built, finances to be raised, and sickness to be conquered and lived with. Sometimes things I've dreamt of have slipped away, like my tenuous grip on sanity.

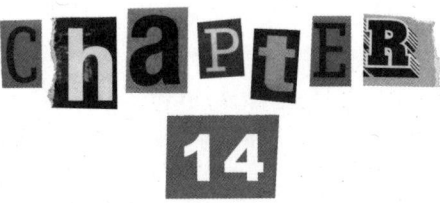

CHAPTER 14

Prometheus unbound

One of the things that got me thinking about writing down my own experiences was the fact that I couldn't find much literature on bipolar mood disorder – besides Kay Redfield Jamieson, whom I worship for writing *The Unquiet Mind*. I think it's the definitive account of bipolar disorder from the point of the person going through it.

Whenever I go to the psychology section of a book store I find hundreds of books on codependency, alcoholism, bulimia, having a bulimic partner and a bulimic aunt, surviving cancer and surviving bankruptcy. Not too much about mental illness. I think that as a society we're somewhat embarrassed about and awkward around mental illness – possibly because psychiatry is such a young profession, possibly because mentally ill people are so unpredictable, and possibly also because of the issue of proof.

Where's the evidence that you're sick? Once, talking to a friend, I mentioned something that had happened while I was in a funk. He said, 'What, you've even given it a name?' He's not an unkind person, just uneducated. I've had friends tell me that I need a life coach to come kick me up the ass and into shape.

Gigi told me a story about a friend of hers, a very successful lawyer, who suffers from anxiety disorder. As this disorder becomes more common, so, too, it becomes more treatable. Being a responsible, self-realised person, Gigi's friend took herself off to the doctor, who put her on Aropax, a very effective anti-anxiety medication. Nobody really was any the wiser. The panic attacks stopped and she was pleased.

Then she decided to take out life insurance. On the form, under medication, she honestly disclosed Aropax. Her insurance was denied. Well, she thought, she didn't need an insurance company like that anyway, and forgot about the whole issue. Then the law firm she worked for promoted her to partner with share options. All they needed was life insurance. Again she was honest. Again her insurance was denied.

Her boss called her into his office to say that without insurance she couldn't become a partner. Her boss had just had a heart attack, but that wasn't seen as a problem. Another of the partners was diabetic, another had a gastric disorder. All that was cool. Smoking was cool. But throw in one panic attack and the corporate world, and society as a whole, shifted nervously away.

For a long time I was ashamed of being bipolar. I perceived it as weakness. I was convinced that if I would just stop feeling sorry for myself, if I could pull myself towards myself and exercise mind over matter, I could take control and expel this 'sickness' from my life. It was only when I accepted it as a part of me that living with the symptoms became more manageable.

In my experience, bipolar people rebel against any sense of imposed order. We're drawn to an external chaos that mirrors the internal one: extreme sports, stressful careers, damaging relationships. We're people with a predisposition to insomnia, so crazy hours attract us. But the behaviour necessary for leading a stable life is the antithesis of all this.

I've grilled myself in the art of living a routine-filled life. I need the canvas of my external world to be tranquil and calm. I need a quiet place where I can seek refuge, away from the bedlam in my brain, and this is only achievable in a predictable, seemingly rather dull existence. It took strength to learn the necessity of these elements, because I felt that I was being robbed of my spontaneity.

I need eight hours of sleep a night, and I need to be in bed and asleep at the same time *every* night. Alcohol doesn't work for me. Exercise is a religion. If I'm exercising a lot, my mood is more robust. Some experts say this has to do with the release of endorphins. Exercise seems to keep a kind of protective wrap around my mood. It's my drug. It makes me high if I do enough of it. I'm no expert on the subject, but the way I've come to understand it is that when you're depressed, your brain stops producing protein. In fact, some of the cells shut down. Sometimes, I can actually feel it happening; I feel myself slipping into a fog of dumbness and dementia.

In a depression, all I can manage are DVDs. Usually a voracious reader, I barely succeed in getting through housekeeping and fashion magazines. I read adverts in newspapers.

I have an aversion to recreational drugs. Mind you, people smoking grass are funny and I enjoy being around them. I love a stoned person. But other recreational drugs frighten me. It's not a rational fear, but a hysterical, instinctive one. Many bipolars go through their lives as alcoholics or drug addicts when, in fact, they're undiagnosed manic-depressives. Robert Downey Junior is my favourite example. I wish I could sweep him away, far from the madding crowd. Have him over for Friday-night dinner and get him some decent medical care. (I suspect this is a fantasy women all over the world share.)

I used to love Obex, a diet pill. It was the only medication that brought me remotely close to the powerful and euphoric state of complete mania. Whenever I felt my elusive mania slipping away, I'd start knocking back the Obex. Eventually I could take as many as six a day and still my low-energy mood would win out over the drug.

Many people, I'm told, have succeeded in turning their perfectly stable state into bipolar see-sawing with enough drug abuse. Getting high on cocaine or Ecstasy, brimming with confidence and energy, is a kind of chemically induced mania. Then, coming down the following day, sleeping it off, waking up paranoid and feeling self-loathing, is all together like a mini bipolar episode, compressed into a couple of days. The notion that anyone would voluntarily do that frightens me. I think drugs detach a person from his or her spirit.

A psychologist once told me that coke closes down your heart chakra. People I know and trust can take a drug and suddenly become weird, alien beings. And it's artificial, so I feel I can't access the person inside. The drug obscures them. I'm too thin-skinned, too vulnerable a being to take drugs. I get scared. I'm so exposed, and the person I'm interacting with is so obscured. And I've done coke in the past, so it's awful to think about. Considering how drug mules carry the stuff, it probably came to me via someone's bum. It then got chopped up, was added to a bit of Ajax washing powder and I snorted it, straight up into my third eye. Gross.

Yet my relationship to my bipolar disorder isn't totally liberated. Sometimes I'll say, 'Oh, I was in hospital because of my thyroid.' Other times I'll overcompensate. 'Hi, I'm Rahla, I'm Jewish, I love popcorn and I'm psychiatrically impaired.'

I have found out this truth: I may think I can jeté across the fondant icing of life, pirouette through pain. But every awkward, clunky feeling I've denied has become a part of me, an organic part of me. Left unattended, it grows like James's Giant Peach. And eventually there's that distinct tap, tap, tapping of anxiety playing percussion in my body. They say that the best thing for panic attacks is a brisk walk. Walk off the adrenaline. And it certainly helps, but not enough. I once saw a psychiatrist who was convinced that I wasn't bipolar but rather had panic disorder. It disorientated me. I think my life has been deformed by the disorder of the day.

Had I been correctly diagnosed at the beginning, I imagine plenty of heartache could have been avoided. For instance, I've been told that, nowadays, if psychiatrists see a hyperactive child, they're alerted to the possibility of bipolar disorder, especially in girls. It is also apparently specific to hyperactivity as opposed to attention deficit disorder (ADD).

Also, I developed what was assumed to be anorexia on two separate occasions. This was brought on by mania. Mania renders you invulnerable to the physical needs normal human beings experience. In the olden days bipolar sufferers died – not because they were depressed, but because they were manic. They died of exhaustion and starvation. Manic people talk, talk and talk. The brain speeds up. Speech speeds up. You know the expression 'raving lunatic'? It's real. We rave about anything and everything.

Manic people write symphonies, read minds, perform heart surgery, control vast corporations, fathom impossible mathematical equations and confidently believe that they can change the world. Preoccupations with inane details like food and sleep don't enter the vastness of the equation. Maybe it's because of all the feelings of false grandeur. You feel you're immortal and you don't need food and sleep to sustain you. Mania is the absolute antithesis of Zen. It's a preoccupation with largesse, fullness and speed, multitasking, places to go to, people to see, things to do.

I used to wake up, eat one Côte d'Or chocolate and then go, go, go, spinning like a whirling dervish through the hurly-burly of my mania, oblivious to physicality. Once, during a manic episode, I hung out with drug addicts. If they were on enough speed they could *just* keep up with me, but the moment they were clean, I had to seek out new entertainment. If only this were a measured commodity. If only it could be handed out in degrees. If only it were sustainable. Inevitably, it runs out. Everything runs out.

When you're manic, you're a million dollars' worth. The projects that I've embarked on, the cash I've spent! In the lobby of a very expensive hotel, I once told a suave foreigner my dream of having an orphanage. I'd found the right building, a hugely impractical rambling old mansion that was most definitely not for sale. I sold the suave foreigner every detail of my preposterous fantasy. I was shocked a few days later when a woman phoned from his office to enquire where the orphanage's trust fund was and how they could go about making a donation.

That particular occasion could have had a comically pleasurable repercussion, but there were others. Oy! The bills, the relationships left in tatters, the physical toll on my body. Not too cool. Not too cool at all.

Bipolar businesspeople are often interesting. A guy I knew seemed to have it all figured out. He lived with his family, who monitored his mood at all times. He opened glamorous businesses – IT companies and impossibly trendy restaurants – kept them going for a few months and then, as his mood was about to crash, he'd sell and clear out.

A girlfriend of mine once found herself in London redirecting traffic. Alerted to her increasing mania, her father flew out to rescue her, only to find her in the middle of winter glamorously kitted out in a strappy sundress and Manolo Blahnik sandals. Often people used to ask her in a patronising tone exactly what it was that she suffered from. When she explained, they'd go, 'Oh wow, I also get down one day and am up the next. I think I've got this bipolar thing too.'

'And do you hear voices?' she'd ask.

Being manic is like being Prometheus unbound or Icarus in free flight. Instead of fearing the sun's rays, you bask fearlessly in its splendid warmth, drawn like a moth to a flame, closer and closer.

The feeling is addictive. Who wouldn't be addicted to such exhilaration? Life! Alive, alive-o! All senses are heightened. Colours are brighter, people become iridescent and the brain is a marvel. It's like being on Ecstasy or cocaine, I guess, but *more* exhilarating, because the feeling is not chemically induced. It's a gift from the gods and you think it will go on forever.

That's why we don't like medication in mania. And here's the bummer: in my experience, medication isn't as good at preventing the lows as it is at hindering the highs.

At twenty, during that first major manic episode, I danced myself into a tornado and felt on top of the world. Skinny and sexy, I convinced a really dim bank manager to give me a chequebook and loan me enough money to go to Cape Town on holiday – with results that make me a bit nervous around a chequebook even today.

The manic episode lasted a couple of months, with cheques bouncing behind me like basketballs. Over the years the debts I've racked up are astonishing. People always trusted me, gave me credit; kind, good people trying to make their way in the world, and I abused them all. From vets to banks to pharmacies, I was indiscriminate. I just consumed and shopped and consumed and shopped my obsessive–compulsive hat off.

Years later my drawers are still packed with white, famous-brand initials on black lacquer lids, black initials on gold boxes, Chanel and Yves Saint Laurent, as shimmery and shiny as the Hollywood sign. I shopped relentlessly until I'd bought double of every available make-up product. It was shocking. It was thrilling. My loving husband worked like crazy to pay off the cosmetic bills alone. It was insane. If I live for another hundred years I'll never run out of lipstick (and I practically sleep embalmed).

Jason used to joke that he could drop me off in a Third World country and within a week the economy would go into a boom. I could buy anything from anyone. When I'm manic, I could buy sand in the Sahara. Why do manic people do this? Why do we need to procure and acquire useless glittering things? More and more meaningless stuff, as pointless as drug addicts determined to get one more fix. Drug addicts go into a space where only the addict and the next fix exist. People exist only to make the fix more accessible, and if they can't do that, then they can piss right off. I've been like that with shopping.

There's a scene in the film *Mr Jones* where the bipolar character, played by Richard Gere, walks into a music store and insists on buying every single piano in the store. Why? It is what it is – mania is not a Zen state of being. There's unbounded consumption of people, of things, of life – just not of sleep or food.

If only the frail human body was designed to sustain this life-style. Maybe the physical exhaustion contributes to the inevitable crack-up. None of us is invincible. It's a cruel illusion played on us by the sickness.

Another aspect of mania is how profligate, thoughtless and irresponsible it is. There's a sense of recklessness that leads to car crashes, a lack of regard for mortality, for life and the feelings of other people. Often the damage to relationships, careers and entire worlds can't be undone. My sister Gigi says that it was only after I was correctly diagnosed that I began to live in the real world, to successfully coexist with its inhabitants.

I was all of twenty-eight – some eight long years after my first manic episode – when the Happy Potter doctor casually announced to me the two words, 'bi' and 'polar'. Separately they're not as ominous as they are combined. Bi can mean so many things. It implies a certain sense of sharing. Polar I associate with Polar Bear ice creams, vanilla-flavoured, coated in chocolate. Put bi and polar together, however, and it's a pretty off-putting diagnosis, so much so that I initially rejected it. This diagnosis came after ADD, hyperactivity, remedial problems, dyslexia, anorexia nervosa and bulimia. As I took in the words 'bi' and 'polar', all those previous diagnoses suddenly seemed, while desperate, at least commonplace.

Princess Diana had made bulimia famous, and really, you hadn't lived if you hadn't experienced the childlike frailty of anorexia. In a funny way, there's a sense of divine control that comes with anorexia. But bipolar, uh-uh. That seemed more like schizophrenia or psychopathy. I'd never really known anyone who had it. Or maybe I had, but they didn't have the T-shirt or drive a car sporting the bumper sticker, so I wasn't aware of it.

I'd always felt neurotic. I still often do – a hypochondriac, a naughty child. Did being bipolar confirm all of these fears? No, altogether this shoe didn't fit. This tiara didn't sparkle. I rejected the diagnosis and returned to my wayward ways: drinking, drugging and crazy living.

Tequila, oh my God, how I loved tequila. Tequila isn't like any other alcohol. People don't just 'like' tequila. No way, it's like Quentin Tarantino; it evokes strong reactions. You don't casually sip on a little tequila over dinner. It's hard-core stuff. It doesn't make you drunk; it makes you high.

When I met Jason, I had a blemish on my right hand from where I used to pour Tabasco sauce. I used to drink a dollop of Tabasco and then follow it with a double tot of tequila. He said that if that's how Tabasco corroded the skin on my hand, imagine what it did to my stomach. God, I loved it; it was the coolest party trick!

How the fact that I was manic, even if only slightly so, eluded the psychiatrist and clinical psychologist I was seeing for so long still puzzles me. My shopping seemed more excessive than that of Imelda Marcos. In my pyjamas at 2 a.m. I'd walk up and down the road, garden secateurs in one hand, spritzer in the other, picking the neighbours' roses. And what did my psychiatric team at the time give me? Antidepressants and Ritalin. Didn't touch sides. If anything, they made me more manic.

Eventually, with the resounding crash of enthusiastic toddlers playing percussion, I collapsed and was forced to go back to the Happy Potter doctor, eating a great stale slice of humble pie and looking more sincerely into the ominous diagnosis of bipolar disorder.

Medicating this disorder is an intricate art form, a balancing act. I have the greatest respect for those practitioners who succeed in getting it right. The human brain is a delicate, vulnerable thing. The chemistry of the mind is like those tiny Russian gymnasts seemingly effortlessly cartwheeling over precariously raised bars.

We take our minds so much for granted and we're so gloriously unaware of the detailed workmanship that goes into a sustained performance. When I'd down a tequila and the effect was so instantaneous, it never occurred to me that something else might be being compromised. I'd sit around with a bunch of friends, motherlessly stoned at 4 a.m., and one of them would say to me, 'Shew, hey, Rahla, you've got to get off those psychiatric drugs, man, they're bad for your brain.' Duh!

I've learnt to respect the magical intricacies of the human mind and psyche and I've learnt to respect the magicians who painstakingly and successfully manipulate the fragile ecosystem of the mind. When things don't work, when our mood is erratic, we're too consumed with self-loathing and anger to consider the possible causes. Maybe it's as much as we can bear, living as we do in such a highly specialised world. We know so much about nothing that we know nothing about everything. We don't take into account the fact that stress goes somewhere, not somewhere out there, but somewhere *in here*.

Even at the peak of my dancing years, I couldn't do the splits. One day my teacher said to me, 'Somewhere in your life you experienced pain and, rather than work through it, you thought if you ignored it, it would go away. Instead it's remained inside and is blocking your body, preventing those muscles from stretching.' I stopped dancing, but a few years later, happily married and generally a more evolved person, I returned to the studio. At the end of my very first class, I almost fell into the splits. I think that my heart was full and my spirit supple. Doing the splits is not merely a physical act.

Often I hear people saying things like, 'I was quite uptight that day, so I took an extra half a Valium,' and I despair for the poor doctor whose formidable task it is to eradicate that person's anxiety.

Medicating the mind is not a hocus-pocus affair. When I was diagnosed with bulimia, I was put on Prozac. It's a great drug and very effective in the treatment of bulimics when administered in high doses. It helped me out of my bulimia, it helped me out of my depression, but I suspect that it also helped me into a full-blown manic episode.

CHAPTER 15

Suicide notes

It's difficult to think about suicide when you're not suicidal, when you're in a garden surrounded by shocking-pink azaleas, scarlet camellias and mauve lavender spikes. The fragrance alone is surely enough to tempt even Sylvia Plath to withdraw her head from the oven. And yet I know better.

That's the funny thing about suicide. It seldom has anything to do with realistic circumstances, with life's true geography. What really happened, how and when and where, is another kind of story. Suicide has its own logic.

Being suicidal is a lingering kind of sickness, one that travels through souls, sometimes passed down from generation to generation. There's a freaky story of a mother hanging herself in the family home on Christmas Eve. Twenty years later, come Christmas Eve, her daughter hangs herself too.

Sometimes, suicide travels insidiously, like a virus. After Romantic poet Thomas Chatterton committed suicide, it became so popular for young love-struck Victorian men to follow suit that his 'life-threatening' book was banned. Copycat suicides are a phenomenon the world over.

Perhaps suicide picks out its victims before they are born, and they're powerless to resist. That's just a weird theory I've cooked up over the years, possibly as a defence against the enemy. Despite all the statistics and doctors' warnings, despite memories of stomach pumps and bandages, I don't see myself as suicidal.

What I do know, sure as the flowers and the glory of the sun, is that when suicide makes a serious, committed call, whatever exists in my life, I answer the phone. Rahla becomes a mere drop of water in the current being pulled inevitably towards the ocean. It's nature, the force of nature.

Ironically, I'm a great lover of life. So was Virginia Woolf, whose infectious, whooping laugh sounded like an owl hooting. I've fought against the demons. I've made serious attempts on my life three times, and each attempt was preceded by days, weeks, even months of despair. People who have a need to kill themselves aren't more cowardly or braver than people who aren't visited by such an urge. They just are.

Back, back, stepping back to when I was a child, visited by the eerie presence of a gnarled old man's face. He was always laughing at me, an ominous, dismissive 'Ha, ha, ha!' Intermittently throughout my life, during panic attacks, driving lessons and falling in and out of love, I'd hear him. He sneered at my achievements and gloated knowingly at my failures. He marked down the days of my life. And he seemed to travel with his partner, Suicide.

Now, though, I imagine they're both far away as I gaze at the old lemon tree draped with baskets of petunias. Any moment now Livicky and Jason will come home and disturb the perfect quietness of the garden. We'll eat pancakes with cinnamon and sugar and shriek with laughter in the undignified manner typical of my family. In the distance kids are playing 'Marco Polo' in their pool and a dog barks as he runs circles around them. Judy Garland sings, 'S-s-s-somewhere over the rainbow', and I know that I will live here, in this wonderful body, in this funny, wobbly, unique body, to a healthy old age.

I know that sometime soon a baby crib will rock among the petunias in the sturdy branches of that lemon tree. And we'll all live happily ever after, because that is who I am. I am of the pink, sparkly, enchanted world of the *Wizard of Oz*. I am one of the lucky few who gets to live over the rainbow. One of the lucky ones who gets away, who gets to survive.

Truth be told, though, Judy Garland was singing exactly the same song in her throaty voice six months ago when all I could hear was the voice of a doped-up, bloated, desperate child.

Poor December. In all its festive innocence it was charged with the responsibility of dispelling a shocking year. It started out well enough in the luxury hotels of Hollywood and New York as Jason and I travelled while he was filming, but rapidly spiralled into misery. We fought with builders over the building of our house, the film Jason had been working on fell through, Gigi decided to take her children and move to New Zealand, I crashed my car, my friend Adam got AIDS and my brother-in-law, Greg, died.

Geg, I called him; Geg, who was aware of me before I met Jason, Geg, who warned his brother that I was wild, that he'd seen me belly-dancing on a table in a restaurant. Later we'd sometimes connect in the crazy world that I inhabit and self-consciously make gestures of friendship and intimacy. Every year he'd bring a birthday cake for me with a Barbie doll perched on top, standing upright like Anna Nicole Smith in a huge pink dress covered in baroque confectioner's roses. I think he delighted in the silliness of it, the silliness of me.

I was so other than he, who was macho to the extreme. Greg was an inspired businessman, a doting father and husband. He was also a wild man, a drug addict, a control freak and a lunatic. He was the Godfather, a builder of empires, a misunderstood child, a misdiagnosed fighter for peace, an in-your-face fighter for the sake of a good fight, and, inevitably, a fellow bipolar.

Greg needs his own book. He's too big and loaded and bloody to write about in a few lines. My story is the one that's about Barbie-doll birthday cakes and how they hold the power to save lives. A fine silver thread that seems to connect our lives as we revolve like unclaimed baggage on an airport carousel, around and around, making patterns and tapestries. But Greg wasn't of the world of the Barbie. He 'got' it, but it wasn't his. He was the suitcase taken home by the wrong owner.

Six months after Greg died I slid into my own floundering process after I went off my medication to try to get pregnant, and went so far as to flounder into a hot, fig-scented bath with a knife.

January the first is not a good day to attempt suicide. Ambulances and hospitals are otherwise preoccupied (ironically, the festive season prolifically churns out its own suicides – people who have a disappointing Christmas). Also, psychiatrists go on family vacations to uncontactable locations.

My fantasy psychiatric institution is populated with songwriters who have wounded eyes. They're all wacky, arty people who are misunderstood and misdiagnosed. In my fantasy psychiatric institution by the sea, there's a fat, smiling nurse from the Deep South who bathes me with a sponge and says, 'Tut-tut, missy, never you mind, you'll get Tara and Rhett Butler back.'

In my fantasy there's always one funny girl who eats copious amounts of candy (she's trying to get off heroin, which she got onto in the first place because her rich parents don't understand her). All the inmates sit around smoking and listening to the solemn songs of Jim Croce, forging bonds of mutual understanding that will outlive our insanity.

In the real institutions, I got abrupt nurses and a hillbilly playing with my hair. Psychiatric wards are marginally better – those wards of crazies within a hospital of normally sick people. Being in these wards is not unlike an aerobics class where you can rest assured that there'll always be people thinner and fitter than you, along with people even less coordinated than you. I may have had festering self-inflicted wounds, but in the room next door was a girl who had signs all over the door instructing staff to 'carefully, thoroughly wash all extremities' before entering her sterile, frequently scrubbed domain.

I developed a life-embracing trick of willing myself back into the world when I got too disappointed. I'd write on my wrist with a permanent marker the names of all the people I loved. For a time it was effective. My psychiatrist was impressed by my ingenuity. He was also impressed by my suicidal tendencies, and accordingly increased the dosage of my mood stabiliser.

But I was miserable. The shame that comes with the guilt that comes with the sadness that comes with the defeat that comes with the desolation of a failed suicide attempt is awful. Once a person has been 'rescued' from the danger of his or her own destructive hand, one assumes that all is well. In fact, the rescued person rarely seems to enjoy the sense of relief felt by loved ones. Well, not in my experience anyway.

December and January were awful months for a girl to be me, and alive. Mind you, Jason wasn't exactly having the time of his life. He had had the romantic experience of finding me poker-faced and bleeding in the boiling, scented water of the bathtub and had had to rush me to hospital. It was the day before his birthday.

Sometimes a depression would descend gradually, giving plenty of warning of its all-encompassing presence and that soon nothing else would be felt. It would be initiated by a sense of inertia, or laziness. A party I was looking forward to attending became a potentially huge ordeal. Next, my routine evening walk with friends would unexpectedly cause panic in the pit of my tummy. Then, leaving the house at all became impossible. Answering the phone grew too troublesome, having to explain the inexplicable misery of my mood.

I'd pick up a book in which I was thoroughly engrossed the previous day and suddenly couldn't fathom the plot. I couldn't remember which character was which, the text became too small and I needed a dictionary to decipher the misplaced meanings of every second word. I'd switch to *Vanity Fair* magazine. Soon the articles would become too long and convoluted. Finally, I just skimmed the pages of women's fashion magazines, barely able to decipher the plot of the *vershtunkende* horoscopes.

Periods of free time would become longer and lonelier. I'd begin to forget vital phone numbers. Recipes would become incomprehensible, containing too many measurements and ingredients. Anything with numbers would become a source of alarm. My deck of tarot cards would present an indecipherable mystery. Even the most menial of tasks would become undoable. Washing my hair, too complicated. How many minutes must the conditioner remain in the towel-dried hair? How would I know when the minutes were finished? One by one, every functioning aspect of my brain would be taken from me. I'd become a catatonic blob, too afraid to venture off my bed, out of my bedroom and into the dangerous, unpredictable domain of my own home.

Then the panic attacks would come, accompanied by blinding migraines. Once again I'd find myself in a miserable heap on the bed as my kindly, calm GP smiled reassuringly, injecting me with Pethidine or morphine, the only drugs that took away the pain. Valium, Ativan and Xanor for panic – glug, glug, glug – deeper I'd fall into the bliss of unconsciousness. Everything would become blurry – the pain, the relentless sadness, people. Less and less light penetrated the velvety darkness of oblivion. Rather like drowning, glug, glug, glug. Relief, blissful relief – until I'd wake up and the cycle would begin again.

Finally, I'd be sitting across a walnut table staring into the compassionate eyes of a doctor who had all the time in the world. And then the dreaded word – relapse.

But sometimes, as now, depression descended with no apparent warning. Crash! and all was darkness in the world. December came with the Crash! Nothing gradual about that descent. One minute I was icing a cake and the next I was locked in the toilet, wrapped in the foetal position, screaming down the neighbourhood. There seemed to be little rhyme or reason, except maybe the season. I'd forgotten to weigh the losses, the disasters and the deaths of the preceding year.

I suppose I'd been thoroughly relishing a mini mania, flying around in a creative whirl of shopping and preparation. Enjoying the familiar feeling of weightlessness, of detachment from the constraints of my physical body. Around September my jeans had started to feel looser. For a while, the behaviour of the people around me appeared unpredictable, sometimes even unkind. I was not going mad. The rest of the world had turned peculiar. And, oh, oh! Move over kidney, heart and lungs, because here come 'The Crazies' – my family, who were moving in for a while.

'The Crazies' and I had been preparing a fantasy birthday party for Jason, to make up for all the past missed birthdays. There were individual scented posies of flowers for each carefully chosen guest. There was special paper on which we were each going to write down New Year's wishes and resolutions. We were going to roll our wishes into scrolls and plant them with violets in the crevices of my garden wall, where they'd blossom and grow. The cake was silver, covered in old-fashioned sugared roses. No expense had been spared. 'The Crazies' and I wrapped presents for each guest.

But on the morning of the party, 1 January 2004, Jason phoned all the guests, apologising and telling them not to come. I lay crying while he cleaned up the miserable carcass of festivities that never took place.

I was hanging on by a fine thread, as fine and delicately made as a spider's web. I became the ugly, dirty fly trapped in the sticky web. I had only one sure way out, one sure way out …

CHAPTER
16

Falling blossoms

George was like a branch of blossoms in an enchanted secret garden behind a high wall. The flowers compel your gaze, their fragrance casts the spell of ancient kingdoms. You can place a branch of blossoms gently in a vase, but it won't last. And if you're rough with it, its blossoms come tumbling down, tumbling down. But then, falling blossoms are a devastatingly, religiously beautiful sight. That was George.

He couldn't possibly have remained on his branch. He had to be adored and appreciated in the spring, because his winters were pure despair. I first met him when I was nineteen years old. It seemed as if George's sole purpose in life was to be fabulous, to be flown around the world drinking pink champagne at breakfast and spraying Chanel No. 5 at passing strangers who took his fancy. He had 'benefactors', fabulously rich people who demanded and sponsored his presence at glamorous parties in exotic places. He was a disco queen, famous in New York, mentioned in Andy Warhol's diaries. He did a rendition of 'Somewhere Over the Rainbow' that could melt a tyrant's heart.

Once, on the promenade in Cape Town, a gust of wind blew up my skirt, exposing my shabby old knickers. Within two days a box of silk La Perla underwear wrapped in tissue paper was delivered to my front door. George wouldn't allow me to expose anything but the most delicate handmade lace.

Of course, I do remember that he drank, and there always seemed to be coke about in his glamorous crowd. Strangely, he was the only person I knew who didn't become vulgar or repellent on coke. To me, in my naivety, even at 4 a.m. in a nightclub lavatory, hopped up on cocaine, George remained as delicate and refined as pink sorbet served in a crystal flute. It was only years later that I learnt the truth: after we'd all called it a night and gone to bed, George would sit up, coked up, all alone on drugs, alcohol and chaos. Party-time over.

Sometimes he'd send me a 'care package' from New York: a box of American trinkets, candy, postcards of Marilyn Monroe, cosmetics and Chanel. I believed he was perfect. He became an artist, doing portraits of New York's rich and famous; portraits as detailed, intuitive and intricate as he was himself.

He ran with a fast crowd. He got into trouble. His fabulousness turned foul. He was diagnosed bipolar. Discovering that he was buried in serious debt (as bipolar people are wont to be), concerned friends bailed him out and brought him back to South Africa. He was a broken-down, drawn, humble shadow of himself.

The medication George was prescribed robbed him of all life

and light. It robbed him of his art and his candyfloss demeanour. He joined a religious sect. They kept him quiet. Then his medication was reduced and modified, and, although he wasn't a laugh a minute, he was more like his old self. He drew magnificently, and he emanated tranquillity and the ironically frothy depth of people who have returned from the dead.

He seemed so well that, at a New Year's Eve party in Cape Town, someone insisted he enjoy just one glass of Moët. Later, someone else gave him a 'little red bomb' (barbiturate), so that he could kick up a heel and relax for old times' sake. He found a 'healer' who succeeded in getting him off his medication.

Before long he was once again the fabulous, irrepressible life force whom everyone had loved all those years before. Some old friends tried desperately to rescue him. Other old friends desperately embraced the glamorous party animal they'd lost for so many years.

He lived out his script. In December 2001, George's sister found him dead in a Donna Summer pool of glitter. I wasn't even remotely surprised. But a part of my heart broke. The rosy tint through which I had enjoyed my vision of the world turned angry amber. The truth is, candyfloss and blossoms don't keep.

When a person I love dies, the harmony of my life is shattered into chaos. I don't feel safe in the world and I'm reminded that we can all lose the people we love most. Death is random. My grand faith in a higher being flounders, and I'm lost. But then I notice the little daily occurrences of my life and I'm reminded about people's innate ability to uplift and understand one another. I believe in humanity and the serenity of the little ecologies we create. Small daily exchanges. The dependable warmth of a checkout lady who shares her life stories with me as she packs my groceries. The neighbour who stretches over her fence every evening to talk nonsense. When my faith in God falters, well, sometimes a more earthly light illuminates. The kindness of strangers, the proverbial 'kind' of humankind, the way we touch one another, unexpectedly, unconditionally. We have a common vein travelling through us all, something universal that makes us understand one another, derive joy from each other.

And God knows, that helps, but it hasn't made it easy. Every time someone I love who has happened to be bipolar has died, I've felt a little more alone in the world. I hear the laughter of the old man in my head becoming more cacophonous, more triumphant and more menacing. He's determined *always* to have the last laugh.

CHAPTER 17

Trawling for Tallulah

My third serious suicide attempt left me with faint, spidery scars on my inner wrists. The lingering characteristic throughout is the rational thinking behind these crazy impulses. At my most suicidal I'm also, in a bizarre manner, at my most rational. Suicide is fantasised about for hours. Plans are meticulously, callously designed and executed without histrionics. I'm deathly calm. There's no light at the end of the tunnel.

Afterwards, I waited for the darkness to lift once again. January 2004 remained bleak. In February, little rays of sunshine began filtering through the despair. Still bandaged but believing myself healthy enough to reproduce, I determined in February, against the advice of the doctors treating me, to go for my first fertility treatment. (Clearly I was thinking that this pregnancy would save me from myself, which is both an egotistical and a stupid way to reproduce.) By this time Jason had convinced my mother to drop her entire world and move to the Cape, where she could take care of me as we attempted, once again, to reproduce with our own DNA.

About a year after the specialists in Johannesburg had told us we'd never have children, I'd been to see another specialist. This time I'd been told that maybe, small, small maybe, we could take Jason's sperm and mix it up in a Petri dish on the outside chance that it might happily go back inside me.

In vitro fertilisation (IVF) is the miraculous scientific intervention of getting babies artificially inside mothers' wombs. It costs a fortune, it is uncomfortable and it isn't always successful. But sometimes it gets a baby where a baby wouldn't otherwise go.

Every day for ten days I got a shot of hormones. They made me retain water and feel nauseous, headachy and hungry. They bloated my body, blemished my skin and fouled my mood. I came to understand that if I was really intent on having a baby, I had to experience this cornucopia of symptoms while my uterus became lined with the gooey stuff babies apparently cling to. Jason had to fork out enormously for the IVF process, whether successful or not. My imaginary child, whom I fondly called Tallulah, apparently felt none of these symptoms.

I remember counting each day until I could have the blood tests to check whether I was pregnant. With only four more sleeps to go, I promised myself that whatever the results were, I wouldn't be entirely unhinged when I heard them. I also promised myself that if I were pregnant, it would be a pregnancy of milk and honey. Still and calm, peaceful and nurturing. Herb teas and classical music. No horror movies or rock music, just calm and quiet. If I were pregnant, I thought, the best thing would be to assemble a bomb and drop it over the noisy neighbours' house, together with a box of homemade fudge and a brief letter of explanation.

It seemed I'd been waiting for Tallulah forever, since the dawn of time. And I do believe all that Nietzschean stuff about the universe conspiring to bring things about. If a person really needs something badly enough, all the energy milling about on God's green earth consolidates to provide it.

The first time I had IVF, the little sea monkey (egg) stayed inside my tummy for just a few days. I looked at the stain in my panties and for the next couple of days thought there had been a mistake. I convinced myself that Tallulah was still there, in spite of the bleeding. Then reality kicked in. I'd known it would probably require more than one shot, but I'd had such a miserable life for such a long time, I wasn't robust enough to handle another disappointment. My heart just about broke.

Tallulah wasn't coming. Oh no. Possibly, she was sensibly squeamish about my recently bandaged wrists, didn't feel that I was suitably prepared. Maybe she had a point. But the failure of the first IVF brought with it a huge sense of disappointment. I'd thought that pregnancy would come to me like a religious miracle, bringing with it relief from the emotional pain of the previous months. With the disappointment came weeks of panic attacks, migraines and misery. Desperate, I considered going back onto all my medication and yet again putting Tallulah on hold.

For a few months it seemed there'd be no respite. My life was wallpapered in misery. Not a twinkle of light could whisper into the impenetrable darkness. I stumbled about in a world of grief, my right foot confusing itself between the brake and the accelerator during a panic attack while driving on the highway; the carcass of my smashed car on a bright Thursday morning. The shadow of sun on the gaunt face of my suddenly aged, sick friend. The thud of sand falling onto Greg's coffin as the finality of his death struck me. The wrinkles that appeared on my own skin, the cellulite that formed to warn me that time was charging on, with or without me. The inevitability of time, and time moving on. How fragile we are, how fragile we are.

Then slowly, slowly, the wallpaper started to bubble, to peel away from the wall of my being, and the natural glow of my world started shining through. The cycle of tragedies seemed to turn, setting the wheel of spring in motion. And once I could discern bits of my life shining through, the desire to start living again started up inside me. After all the sorrow, I had a good year. I enjoyed a few months of good health. Not a single migraine, panic attack or crying germ. I was miraculously stable.

I didn't make the mistake of thinking the bliss would last forever, and I savoured every minute. I knew that darkness could descend *manyana, manyana, manyana*, but in the meantime I had a mighty fine window period.

And it's through those precious window periods in the illness that I get to look out at the sea, at the world in all of its rose-tinted loveliness. I have the rich moisture of laughter, not the desolate dry landscape of sadness. I peer through the obscure veil masking real life and find that my mood, if nothing else, is fertile. Singing again: 'I can see clearly now, the rain is gone ...'

With my health and my beloved husband in my arms, I wondered what more a girl could ask for. Oh yes, there was definitely more. If the cupcake could be in the oven, if I could finish writing my *vershtunkende* book and if it could be marginally readable— Oh, and I wondered aloud to God, would it be asking too much if I could get the pimple on my forehead surgically removed?

The time drew closer, the days grew longer as winter started to shift its miserable cloud and spring started peeping in. The waiting became more agitating. I picked a twig of flowering white-and-pink jasmine, making my bedroom smell of the swimming pool at the back of my parents' garden.

Years and years of poolside memories flooded back – little children leaping gleefully off Daddy's shoulders into the cool water. David as a teenager, patiently coaxing me out of the shallow end and into the brave new world of doggy paddle in the deep end. My best friend Brian and I rescuing 'drowning' ladybirds and placing them like precious trophies on the burning poolside slate to dry out. The slate on which we wrote secret messages like a magical blackboard, where our words would instantly vanish, evaporated by the glorious Highveld sun. Jonty shouting 'Marco!', Gigi shouting 'Polo!' and my first dog, Lolly – the black-and-tan miniature dachshund that I didn't yet know was mortal – running frantically round and round the pool after children who couldn't keep still until, desperate to be a part of the game and overexcited, he took a corner too quickly and slipped into the churned-up water. Pnina leapt in to rescue him and we wrapped him up like a hot dog in our towels.

Memories came back, catching me unawares. The smell and taste and excitement of smooching boyfriends and getting stoned in the springtime. The smell of adventure and summers that greedily seemed to go on and on for all the days of our blissful childhood. A sexy, lingering smell.

I wondered what Tallulah's childhood summers would smell like to her. The smell of her godmother's Fracas perfume and home-made chicken soup, the smell of her godfather's faraway lands and great spiritual conquests. The smell of the seaside and watermelon eaten as you splash in the water of the swimming pool, leaving pink trails of juice and pips floating over the rim. Perhaps her world would be all about spangled ballet tights and the delicious, cherished smell of the nape of her daddy's neck as she sat on his lap in the strange film-editing suite.

A secret world of darkened cinemas and dreams captured on celluloid after the frenzied magic and chaos of film sets. Music and dancing and dressing up and watching one brilliant film after another all her childhood long. Or a world of grubby fingers digging into the earth and planting, planting and weeding with her mother who loves gardens but can't garden for toffee. Would her world smell of mountain climbing with her *safta*, Livicky, or wearing make-up with her Aunt Pnina? All the people – I wondered at all the people she might choose to become.

Then someone recommended a reflexologist, who recommended a health store, who recommended a professor of acupuncture for fertility treatment. Thus I found my Pokémon Professor of light, life and instant relief.

While I was explaining that I wanted to get pregnant, he said to me, 'Show me tongue, please?' Examining my tongue, he said, 'But you have headache, no?' Headache indeed! My head felt as if bands of invading soldiers were banging away at the bone. 'I can put needle for headache?' A needle, yes; pins, needles, anything to relieve the pain, I said, and twenty minutes later I walked out with no pain, no anxiety and very little depression to speak of. I had started that first consultation a murky shade of green and ended it rosy-cheeked and healthy.

At a later session, the Pokémon Professor looked again at my tongue and said, 'Your body no like sugar.' No, my body doesn't, but I adore it and was consuming three packets of candy a day. He put needles in my ears and, whoosh, no candy cravings! He then put a needle into my ear in a special spot named the *Shen Men*, the gateway for the spirit. Suddenly my spirit was released, flying freely in a toxin-free universe. The candy must have been blocking the gate.

After my second IVF treatment, Jason accompanied me for the egg harvesting. I wore china-blue-and-white pyjamas with a pink pashmina, but the nurse who administered fabulous drugs (premeds, Dormicum, local anaesthetic and the likes) insisted I change into a regulation calico nightie with tie-ups at the back. The Stork Doctor needed easy access to my fanny.

Jason and I got into an altercation about my care-package requirements. I wanted loads of fresh flowers, wheat- and sugar-free vegan carrot cake and hanging crystals, convinced that Tallulah wouldn't make an appearance unless she saw evidence of a fragranced, feminine, magical universe. Or else she'd come out as a boy – not Tallulah, but Tom. Jason thought I was being too demanding. But mid-discussion, the world started going glug, glug, glug and taking on a sublime, marbled hue. Too late I remembered how desperately I needed a bikini wax … glug, glug, glug …

When I came to, Livicky appeared with a miserable handful of tatty pink-and-red roses and Jason returned from the supermarket carrying white chrysanthemums. Twelve years together, and he handed me chrysanthemums. I loathe chrysanthemums. There's something so smug and provincial about them. I packed in two carrot cakes and smiled patronisingly at him.

Slowly the world came back into focus. Five eggs. They'd harvested two fat, healthy eggs and three *verlep* ones. Five eggs! Each egg could divide into two. Imagine, ten fat healthy Xenopouloses. Satisfied, I anticipated phase two. With some luck the sperm had been successfully defrosted and were joyfully frolicking in a Petri dish with the five fat eggs, making friends and discussing plans for their future existence.

Someone told me an amazing theory: When the sperm and egg connect, there's just half an hour in which the precise personality, the life choices, the very DNA thumbprint is established. I find that extraordinary.

On the surface, I suppose such talk could be misconstrued as anti-abortion (I loathe the term pro-life), but I don't think it is at all. Those little beings made their own decisions about whether or not to be born now. God willing, not every single one of the eggs presently gadding about was going to multiply and be born in nine months' time. They were just play-acting the different options available to them.

'I intend to come into the world with an unsightly harelip. Then, after extensive, traumatic surgery, my harelip will be successfully altered into an unusual, striking birthmark and I shall become a world-famous underwater ballerina. Just kidding. I'm not actually incarnating this time round!' And so it was, I imagined, role-playing in the Petri dish.

I returned to the hospital sixty days later. I hoped Tallulah's tadpoles would be successfully transplanted from the Petri dish into my womb. With luck, one of them would like the sounds, smells, tastes and textures therein and park off inside me for the next nine months. Straightforward, really. Reproduction. Nothing to it.

The Stork Doctor, our fertility expert, called and said three of the eggs had successfully germinated – a potential three Xenopouloses. Yikes a doodle dandy! He told me to insert a vaginal suppository every morning, the vaginal pills every evening and not to worry if any of the progesterone leaked. Frankly, I think being a heroin addict is probably more dignified than making babies.

I was terribly concerned about the responsibility I might be taking on of bringing another deranged person into the world.

Chances of chemical imbalance are high for Tallunks, pretty high. She's got it bad on her father's side and, well, there's some rather crazy DNA coming from her mother's genes.

But in those weeks of waiting, with needles in my ear and progesterone in all manner of places, I found myself just sitting on our deck, watching the ships go by. All was well in my world. I had three eggs, germinated, waiting to be transferred into my tummy. I had Jason carrying in a silver tray with my breakfast-in-bed kisses. I had my dachshunds, Taxi and Capote, languishing at the foot of my bed like a pair of furry, copper-coloured mitts. I had the sound of the sea faintly at my window, and the ancient smell of the ocean lacing itself around the scent of the fresh stargazer lilies keeping watch by my bed. No more deadly fig-scented baths for me; banish the thought. No more the fragrance of a mood that implores with a sinister beguiling calling. I was far more robust.

CHAPTER 18

Myself, I've chosen. I chose eleven years ago, on a spring night in Johannesburg, when the air was heady with the smell of jasmine. The world shook that night, a love so great, a meeting so intense that the universe trembled.

That was what got my attention initially, the shaking of the earth. I looked down from my candyfloss bed in my Turkish-delight universe to see what minor quake had occurred on earth. When I found the source of the vibration, my decision was instantly made. I made my choice with as much urgency as they made theirs. Naturally, fool mortals that they are, they assumed the shaking of the earth was imagined, not the real thing it is.

The artist James Jacques Joseph Tissot painted me in 1877, oil on wood. The painting's called 'Hide and Seek'. I'm enchanting, entirely irresistible. Golden curls frolic around the perfection of my face, defying the satin bow that tries to secure them. I'm playing on a Persian carpet wearing a Victorian silk frock. Great big orange bows fall at my shoulders and around my waist. You can just see the heel of my shiny black shoes.

My cheeks are like two dimpled toffee apples, and my mouth, at the age of three, is already set in what will be its lifelong, profane pout. In front of me is a ball. I'm looking at it, smiling to myself. The sofas are covered in sumptuous fur and silk brocades. Thick velvet curtains fall languidly across the windows.

My two beloved boys are always with me, but only I can see them. From everyone else, they hide.

In the painting, my friends peek at me from behind screens and ornaments. My gentle governess, Tatiana, reads the paper. She's been with our family since I was born and will remain with us until my own daughter is born in twenty years' time. As my daughter grows up, Tatiana will pass the raising of infants on to her own child.

You can't see my mother in this picture, because she's in the parlour making lemonade squeezed from fresh lemons from her own tree. Dashes of colour flash from the garden through the windows and the French doors.

I'm like a smiling Buddha, or Oscar Wilde's Happy Prince, frolicking in the gardens of ignorance. Everything my senses happen upon is intoxicating.

Many a lonely night I find myself weary from gazing at the earth and waiting for them to be suitably prepared for my birth. Then I'm tempted to join the boys in Atlanta, where they are going to live. But then I fly through skies of laughing stars, reverberating with the laughter of happy princes and long-lost relatives to the National Gallery of Art in Washington and dwell on that picture, admiring my next life. Mind you, I get confused; it could have been a past life. Either way, Atlanta's not in the picture. I've got it all worked out. I can wait. All these years of waiting will one day be worth it when I'm the child of that love affair.

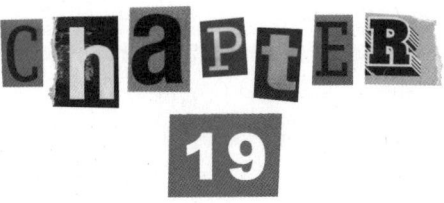

CHAPTER 19

The sea monkey moves into the tummy

I used to imagine Jason's brother Greg and my father in heaven with Tallulah, teaching her important life lessons. Then, once she was inside the Petri dish, I assumed she'd said goodbye to them. I can't picture the ghosts of old souls swimming about a Petri dish with a bunch of tiny eggs; it would be preposterous.

Poor child, if that's the case she'll think all her relatives are barking mad. She'll think violent mood swings are a normal aspect of human life. On bad days it seems like vanity, wanting to reproduce while knowing that my child may suffer as I have. Yet it needn't end in tears. Psychiatry is constantly advancing. We're so much more informed – as a species, as a couple. We've learnt the benefits of gardening, yoga, acupuncture, aromatherapy, diet, abstinence, routine, structure and sleep hygiene. Oh yes, we have many tricks at our disposal.

I read somewhere that doctors will soon be able to pronounce on a baby's mental health before it's born. Mothers could decide to terminate, lest they continue the cycle of madness. What then of Van Gogh, Ted Turner, Virginia Woolf and Stephen Fry? What if Mary Shelley hadn't been visited by a strange madness that became a metaphor for illness in her novel *Frankenstein*? Naturally the world would have fewer suffering people, but it would also be less ravishing. All of us crazy, wonderful types would become extinct, and that seems quite improper.

There must be a reason for all the insanity. We sing a rainbow. We see the whole of the moon. We teach people to be vulnerable, to ache, to plunge into the turbulent river of life. Sickness slows mankind down and teaches us to stop and take care, to nurture one another. How tender, how fragile we are.

I'd like my baby to be aware. Even living here on this bewitching tip of Africa, I'd like her to know that suffering is an intrinsic element of the human condition. I'd like her to cry when she hears Kiri Te Kanawa and José Carreras singing, 'There's a place for us, somewhere a place for us...'

In their profound humanity, I hope those words can touch and transport her to an awareness of the fragility in which people are stirred and suffer so as to create art and beauty. Maybe she'll never make head girl or have straight glossy hair, but she'll sing a rainbow.

Lying in bed the night before the last insemination, I thought that maybe it would be the last time I slept with an empty womb for the next nine months. What a spectacular thought. Well may Kiri Te Kanawa sing, well may the almond tree blossom in the middle of winter.

In the morning, I was in the pink: pink-and-red paisley pyjamas, pink pashmina, pink nails and dark glasses. I was stylishly attired for the occasion of Tallulah's implantation. I waited with the nurse and the Stork Doctor for the lab assistant to bring the 'sea monkeys' up from the lab. I was feigning nonchalance, with my legs up in stirrups, while the doctor smiled encouragingly and a bit awkwardly. The nurse also smiled encouragingly, and a bit awkwardly.

'Don't worry the lab, nurse, my eggs will walk here on their own. They're very advanced, you know,' I volunteered for no apparent reason. Nurse and doctor laughed awkwardly. Patiently I waited for the eggs to come up from the lab and for the bliss of the pre-med to kick in. In case the nurse and the doctor weren't yet convinced that I was barking mad and unfit for motherhood, I felt compelled to tell them the story of the medical student transporting a hand.

'My father and the hand. The young intern was late; he was perpetually late. Some people thought this contributed to his charm. Nonchalantly he whistled through downtown Johannesburg of the late forties. It was full of the glamour and cheek that follow wars. Each heart had a story to tell. The girls, with their perfectly nipped-in waists and white gloves, felt a need to fall in love now that the men were home, no longer abroad, fighting. The men were softening back into society, yet not impervious to the splendour of being alive after a world war.

'Everything was appealing and exciting, including the young intern walking with his jolly friend. They crossed the road from the medical school. In his pocket, the friend carried a human hand they'd just finished studying. An old lady wearing a straw hat covered with flowers stood in front of her broken-down car. Spotting the dashing interns, she enquired, "Excuse me, could one of you gentlemen lend me a hand?" Looking at his friend, Daddy said, "Don't do it, old boy, don't do it." But his friend laughed. "Come on, an opportunity like this comes once in a lifetime." And bowing graciously low as he offered the hand, he said, "Madam, would this do?" With which she fainted.

'When she picked herself up, she marched off to lodge a complaint with the disciplinary board, and Daddy's friend found himself expelled from medical school and seeking a new career.'

There was an awkward silence.

With no more stories to tell, I began to feel the tap, tap, tap of drugs as bliss began to knock at my brain. The lab assistant arrived with the sea monkeys in a plastic cylinder. They looked like a roll of Glad Wrap. Tap, tap, tap. Glug, glug, glug. 'Don't worry, Mrs Xenopoulos, this won't be too painful. It's just like a big Pap smear.' Oh good, and I'm such a fan of a big Pap smear.

It was 22 July, and twenty-two is a good number. It's a feminine number, and in the tarot it's the number of the Fool, which is unconditional love. I felt sure it was a good day for the sea monkeys to go into my tummy.

The Stork Doctor and Pokémon Professor had both advised me to stay in bed for ten days. I listened to Pachelbel's *Canon*. I wished I hadn't rushed through reading *Mrs Dalloway* so quickly. Then I would have been curled up in bed with Pachelbel, paisley pyjamas, dogs, Virginia Woolf and sea monkeys transforming themselves into Tallulah.

The first day I was afraid to wee. What if I weed one out? Oy! And what if all three grew and we had triplets? Jason said, 'I'm warning you, if you have triplets I'll feed only them, not you!' His editor joked that if we had three, she'd keep the runt. Jason said, 'Why stop at one? She could take two. In fact, she's welcome to all three, and we'll just borrow them. Weekly visitation rights.'

Sitting at home, I could barely glimpse the horizon, just the charcoal clouds welling up with rain above the ocean, which was good for the garden. I knew if it rained, my big orchid would flower – a magnificent miracle. 'You hear that, Tallulah?' I whispered. 'Your very own orchid clump, next to the camellias, under the lemon tree.'

Thankfully, the rain slowed me down, making me calmer about being in bed. It's a drag, staying in bed. I can never relax until my environment is perfect: the right fragrance wafting through the room, the right flowers in the right vase next to the bed, which has the softest linen, with enough rainbows dancing through the perfection. And then I'll notice that the window is dirty or that the little Buddha is askew, and I'm up again.

I suppose lying in bed always takes me back to being in a funk, too depressed to get up. It's difficult, being sick. It makes one self-obsessed. There's a constant need to keep assessing symptoms and focusing inwards, internalising, analysing the most inane details of daily occurrences. Doctors, friends, family, healers and trainers are looking to detect changes. Everything in the world shouts out, 'Me, me, me!' For me, the worst thing about sickness, particularly depression and mania, is the loneliness.

These are not experiences easily shared, but my dog Capote had a freaky sense of solidarity with me. He sat by my side constantly, and sometimes alerted Jason to the dip in my mood, whining as if in severe pain. Uncannily, regardless of whether I was in Joburg or Cape Town, Capote would get sick the very day I was checked into hospital and recover the day I was discharged. If I went on a regular vacation, he was fine.

The isolation is terrible. I'm almost compelled to keep journeying inwards, hashing and rehashing the details of the day, the miserable experiences too bleak to share with anyone leading a normal life. Doctors become like religious mentors and I hang desperately onto their every explanation. I have so little contact with the outside world that it begins to seem as though this misery in which I exist is the only life possible. Silly details are amplified irrationally. In my attempt to protect people from the tedium of my mood, I try not to see friends, with the result that I become more self-obsessed. Sick people are in constant danger of becoming small-minded. It's worse on grey days, as if my internal weather mirrored the tones of the outside world.

Waiting for Tallulah to find a comfortable spot in my tummy, I lay in bed, writing, and listening to Jason and Livicky making lunch. She was laughing her hat off. Her laughter almost drowned the racket coming from the neighbours' drumming downstairs. It almost drowned out the sound of the waves crashing in a storm outside.

It was difficult to stay entirely immobile. I fed the fish, threw out a bit of snail bait and snipped violets. I watched the ships go by, waiting for my baby to settle in. I asked the Pokémon Professor if he could diagnose her on my tongue. He said it was too early. After ten days he'd be able to tell from my pulse if I was pregnant or not. But he was adamant I couldn't continue acupuncture through pregnancy. I thought, if necessary, I'd camp outside his surgery. He could take out a court order, but I'd be like an obsessive stalker, immune to rejection.

CHAPTER 20

Tallulah sings her rainbow

Now that my departure is becoming more imminent, the boys become increasingly unsure about our separation. In some way or other we've been together for centuries. Of course, I'm also scared. The geographical divide between us will be vast: Atlanta to Cape Town isn't a mere hop, skip and a jump. It could happen that we go through our whole lives never crossing paths, never meeting, always feeling a dull emptiness in some uninhabited region of our psyches.

Tonight we waltzed above the earth, an irresistible pas de trois. Three little angels we were, a hiss of white chiffon, lost in time and space, we leapt, Strauss's 'Blue Danube' resounding through the atmosphere. We jetéed forty times, from raining cloud to raining cloud. Finally, we struck perfect arabesques for the birds and angels to see. Oh, I shall miss those two.

We've been conspiring about a way for them to join me in my new life in Cape Town. Mind you, I think Rahla and Jason might get rather a shock should I pop out accompanied by an entire kindergarten!

But we have this enchanted spell we've carried with us in our pas de trois *across the centuries. I can't imagine living an entire life without them.*

Naturally we haven't always been siblings. During the Spanish Inquisition we were lifelong friends. I was a Muslim silversmith, and the boys were a pair of Jewish craftsmen, all forced to flee Toledo. During the Russian Revolution we were aristocrats and had to flee again, this time from the Bolsheviks. During the gold rush I was their mother, and we had a circus travelling the country, but heavens, were they wayward sons! And there was I, a mother, a trapeze artist and fortune-teller with two wild boys to care for. Needless to say, we never did strike gold. But we had a fine old time.

I've got this yucky feeling that Rahla will have a natural birth. The last time I was born it was via Caesarean — so much simpler. I came out stress-free and as pretty as a peach. After a natural birth I'll be as wrinkled as an ooold man. Then I'll have half a lifetime to smooth and straighten out before starting to wrinkle up all over again. But whichever way I'm born, this will be my most enchanted lifetime. I've waited to live this particular life for a thousand years.

CHAPTER 21

Hillbillies, Godot and distant siblings

The Pokémon Professor assured me that everything would be hunky-dory without his treatment. He insisted that most of the points he used on me are contraindicative to pregnancy. Imagine poor Tallulah writhing about inside my tummy like the artist formerly known as Prince in her desperate attempts to avoid being punctured by little copper needles. Pokémon Professor and his wife advised me to sit tight and not be active. So the Western doctor and the Eastern doctor concurred. I was pretty much bed-bound with naught for comfort but my *schmutsik* dogs, neroli candles, Virginia Woolf and a pile of notebooks full of pages as empty as the Sahara Desert.

I painted my nails a weird pearly pink. It reminded me of a scene in a film I saw a long time ago. I may embellish here and there; my recollection may not resemble the original at all, so I apologise to the filmmakers if I bastardise their masterpiece.

Here's the scene: Two trailer-park hillbilly dames are hanging out in a diner in deepest, reddest, redneck middle-America. One is in the throes of what appears to be a severe existential crisis. Her boyfriend has dumped her, leaving her homeless and knocked up, with five no-good children, his gambling debt and an empty bottle of rum. Her own health is failing along with her looks. Her mother, the bitch, is dying. Her father is an alcoholic, and her cat, the one entity on this black earth ever to love her, has just drowned. Is life worth living at all?

The friend raises her head from her fried green tomatoes and rhubarb tart, flicking the split ends of her fringe out of her eyes, and says, 'Honey, you know, whenever I'm feeling real, real bad, I paint my fingernails and my toenails a real purty pink. That way, every time I look down, I remember I'm doing jus' fine – how can anything be bad when I have such real purty nails?'

I think of this movie moment whenever well-meaning buffoons volunteer this type of counsel to me, the 'Honey, just pull up your socks, cheer up, look on the bright side, I wish I had your life, maybe you just need to see real suffering, maybe you need to go for a brisk walk, you don't have cancer you know, you need to just snap out of it, stop dwelling, don't believe the labels' kind of advice.

People get mad if you laze about crying when you don't actually have anything physically wrong with you. I've been told that manic depression has a higher fatality rate than cancer. But I'm not climbing on a soapbox – I'm just giving chirpy-chunky-cheerful manicure advice.

I applied an aspect of it to Tallulah. The colour of my nails was such a preposterously juvenile pink that I was betting Tallulah would be drawn, if not to me, then at least to my nails. I knew she'd be annoyed when she discovered that in real life my nails are very rarely painted and, when they are, it's a rather pitiful, chipped, smudged, ebony affair.

I was relieved during the blissful moments when my Navajo neighbours weren't making any tragic attempts at music or power-drilling one another into stupefaction. Some days, all was well in my world and God was in His universe. Everything was pastel, powdery perfect.

I felt sure that Tallulah was gently slumbering in my tummy, soothed by Bach's ethereal *Air on a G String*. In a way I felt relieved that Jason didn't have a movie in production. I'd have gone mad hanging around the house looking at the same splendid view every day while he was out there at four in the morning, eating indigestible food and shouting, 'Action!' I was starting to feel as though it were ten thousand years since we'd been on set. But for all the talent and vision in the world, if you can't hang around *waiting*, you amount to nothing in show business.

So we waited. For film finance, for the sun to set majestically, for Tallulah to arrive, for the garden to establish itself, for Godot to fail to appear. Oh, what an awful lot of waiting is involved in being alive.

When an architect friend was designing our house, I told him, 'I don't want any colour at all, because when the inhabitants of a home have such colourful personalities, you dare not rival them with pink cushions. They'll feel upstaged, which will never do!'

My family, the family that Tallulah is hopefully going to be part of, have always found one another entertaining and clever. The drag of it is how dispersed we are. What is it with Jews and wandering? Pnina at least is in Cape Town, returned from Europe, ever so

157

perfectly glamorous, gorgeous, talented and funny. But David is in Israel, Jonty is in Johannesburg with his heart in Greece, Gigi is in New Zealand, and Jason works in Johannesburg and lives in Cape Town. Like the lost tribe, we're scattered and flung to the four corners of the earth. Is this a South African condition? The Jewish tradition? The modern way? What's with us all?

We've become quite casual about families being divided, but it seems unnatural. We grow up with people who shape our personalities. We're trained to believe that, like it or not, siblings are always around. Then, boom! This one is here and that one is there. No more togetherness.

But children bring us back together. They create new communities out of existing ones. Pnina has chocolate that will miraculously grow out of Tallulah's ears, just as it grew out of mine when I was a child. The *Madeleine* books Livicky read to us when we were children wait patiently for her to read them to Tallulah. Far and wide, the cycles continue; we all go round and round.

I want to plant roses and jasmine in the garden, so that even if Tallulah goes away, she'll come home, as we always do, to the smells and traditions of our childhood.

CHAPTER

22

The stars below me twinkle like jewels draped on a purple carpet. The moon clears a path, illuminating Atlantic Avenue through the blue-black ocean. Twinkle, twinkle little star, how I wonder what you are.

Can we wish on the same bright star as Rahla? The second star on the right, the one that goes straight on till morning. It's a great big star; I'm sure she can also see it wherever she may be. If I wish on it, and she wishes on it, then surely our dream will come true?

I've been wishing on that bright star since God was a boy, just wishing and dancing. So many lives have been offered to me but I've kept on, holding out steadfast for this one. If I stand really still, with my hand on my little belly, I can just about count the flaps of the buttercup-coloured wings of the butterfly that lives inside my tummy.

It's not that I mind being here. This is the heavenly pit stop. We come here between lives to refuel, to take stock and reflect on our most recently passed lives and meditate on the ones to come.

Some people just keep gravitating towards one another and finding one another life after life after life (like me and the boys), but the only thing that's really for keeps is the soul. Each time we're born we have so many new things to learn, so many lessons to complete, it's only natural we're inclined to keep the same people around us.

Often there's unfinished business with specific people and it's not always a pretty affair, but if you don't work through the issues, you have to carry them around with you from one lifetime to the next. It weighs you down, making the soul heavier and heavier, like poor Count Dracula's. 'Try not to die before you've finished all your business this time round': that's the best advice I ever got.

Perhaps the best you can hope to do is to devote yourself to people with whom you have good contracts and try to avoid the ones with whom you've got bad business. The way to judge who's who in your karmic creations is to ask yourself, 'Does this person bring out the me in me that I love?'

If you pay attention and listen to the fast or faltering beat of your heart, it's generally a very clear yes or no. Not a lot of grey in that area. The memories of other people who've crossed your path are imprinted in your soul – not written down, of course; more like fine, scarcely visible fingerprint drawings.

Here we carry our souls around with us all the time. Mine is in a silk mermaid's pouch, attached to my wrist with a daisy chain.

The last thing you do before you go to sojourn inside your mommy's tummy is to pop your soul into your mouth like a giant vitamin pill. After you've swallowed it, it remains inside you throughout your lifetime. So you'd better make pretty darn sure you've got a good soul, 'cos it's the only thing you have forever and ever. If it's a little off-colour, you need to try hard to clean it up, otherwise it gets smelly and festers inside like the alien living inside Sigourney Weaver in Alien. *Of course, if you've got a good soul, it's just like swallowing a bunch of rose petals.*

The more lives you live, the lighter your soul becomes. That's why mine is suspended by a mere daisy chain. Maybe this time I'm not making the easiest choices; maybe I'm picking up some weird genes and I'm going to end up stark raving mad, but who gives a hoot? I'm going to have a grand old time and I'm going to be a magical conduit of love.

We don't go into lives ignorantly. We don't happen upon people and just pop out of their unsuspecting tummies. Sometimes it takes years and years of God's planning and our deliberating. Our options are explained to us and we make informed decisions. There's nothing haphazard about the relationships we have in this world. We can't predict the precise details of our lives, but we do have an idea of the risks we're taking and the dreams we may have.

I've grown bored of listening to all the warnings about the dangers of bipolar disorder. They say 90 per cent of people who suffer from the sickness have a close relative who suffers from some mood disorder or other and having one bipolar parent gives a child a 10 to 30 per cent chance of becoming bipolar herself. And they don't stop trying to frighten me with stories about bipolar mothers.

Fine, I'm choosing really special godparents in case I need extra love and attention if Rahla goes off the rails. I've got grown-ups ready to make extra school lunches and give lifts to and from extramural activities. People to explain to me why my mother is hiding under her dressing table for no apparent reason. And lest I forget, one in every five people with bipolar disorder will commit suicide, and of course the rate of alcoholism and drug abuse is three times higher than it is with other people. Nevertheless, all my bags are packed and I'm ready to go, just like the melodic refrain from a seventies song. I keep telling all the busy-body angels, even God, that I know exactly what I'm doing, and I'm going to have the life of my life!

With or without the genetic disorder that has lived quite happily in the bodies and souls of my new family for generation upon crazy generation.

If you catch a crying germ as a little girl, you can't stop crying and you have to hope and pray that you don't cry all the water and even the blood out of your body, leaving you a dehydrated old desert wasteland with not a mirage in sight. The doctor sometimes punctures you with needles to stop the crying, otherwise he gives you a 'special penicillin treatment' for the aching heart. If, on the other hand, you get 'wings', you just keep on wanting to fly and fly, higher and higher. Close to the sun you soar, and you just hope that your wings don't melt, and your feet don't stumble while walking on the moon. But sometimes the doctor can also give you 'special penicillin stuff' to help you land back on earth.

Of course, the boys still pretend they think I'm making a crazy choice, but I tell them that an animated soul in a dull life is a dangerous thing. It's a wild card, always saying inappropriate things at inappropriate times. A lively soul can become so bored that it starts doing re-ee-ee-ally nutty things. I just don't imagine that a life in Atlanta, with or without the boys, can contain or accommodate nuttiness, so I'll be off to the tip of Africa.

They keep on reminding me about this crazy artist we once knew in France. At the time we were prostitutes, leading a frightful existence. One day the artist came and tried to pay me for services rendered by offering me his ear. He just took a shaving knife and lopped the ear off his head. The boys freaked out, but I rather liked the artist and the funny, warped way he had of seeing life. Simple scenes that you or I might take for granted he painted in magical, swirling colours. He seemed to see the world through the eyes of his sickness, and it made mundane things exciting and wondrous. After his death he became quite famous.

One day, he'd be the busiest, happiest man in the world, frenetically painting away as if he knew his time was running out. Next day he'd be an inert lump of misery unable to make himself a cup of tea. We never knew what was wrong with him, but we did try to look after him.

Nowadays people are cleverer than they were then. It's not like past centuries, less humane and caring, when people with bipolar disorder generally died of exhaustion and starvation during bouts of mania or else got locked away in unsympathetic institutions to sit out the depression all alone. That won't happen to me. I'm going to live in a lovely home looking onto a lemon tree in the little garden.

But que sera, sera, whatever will be will be, the future's not ours to see … as Doris Day once sang. I'll take the downs with the ups and long live the in-betweens. It's going to be just dandy, and if those ragamuffins could come along, it would be even better. I'll begin my life sheltered from the storms in a green bay of the Cape under a flat-topped mountain with a floating cloud that comes and goes.

It's drawing nearer now. Each day it seems more certain. The doubts that plagued me two months ago have been gobbled up and swallowed by my exuberant enthusiasm. I see Rahla's face more vividly than those around me up here. I can hear my father's thoughts, travelling faster than the speed of light through his active mind. I look at them both and wonder: What will I inherit from whom?

Will I inherit his eyes and her laugh? Or maybe my grandmother's laugh? Please, please God, at the risk of sounding picky, could I dance like her and not like him? I'd really appreciate just a bit of his brain; he's got such a dashing brain. I'll be able to cut through all the foolishness of life. Then there are the aunts, uncles and grandparents. Won't it be a thrill if I inherit my maternal grandmother's poise and my paternal grandmother's figure?

Now I sit up at night eating hot chocolate sauce on rye bread and weighing up all the options. I study the various genetic providers, and naturally I'm inclined to mix in only the more appealing ingredients. My mother's lousy vision I've left out of the equation. As for the madness, well, kindness transcends that. I've been alive for an awful number of lifetimes and I can

163

tell you that if the kindness is strong enough, it counters the Crazies most days. The Crazies are fierce animals, but kindness helps you to understand the wild beasts.

Today I looked at my boys while we were playing in the crystal rainbow forest and I could hardly see them. They were just a silhouette of rainbows, almost a smudge. I didn't tell them, but I had a feeling my time here is growing shorter and shorter. I won't be playing in the rainbow forest for much longer. Even if the boys are coming with me, I'll start losing their images as we all metamorphose into human children.

Dear me, they're probably not expecting the boys in Cape Town, whereas in Atlanta they've been praying for them. Whatever happens, somewhere along the way we'll meet again – don't know where, don't know when, but I know we'll meet again some sunny day.

Preparing to leave is rather like packing a satchel for the first day of school – so much anticipation and excitement. If I forget anything, my fruit juice or my pencil sharpener, why, it seems like I'll just die. That first day of school, those six hours, seem to present themselves to a child's delirious brain as the final six hours of life. The opportunity to come home and pack again will never again present itself. This is my only God-given opportunity to get it right.

That's how I feel now, galloping about, disrupting the tranquillity and peace of the place. Trying to capture ideas and faces, trying to catch important details and memories in a butterfly net so that I can pop them in my pouch and they'll be available as déjà vu experiences throughout my long, funny life. Not that I've got such a lot of space in my little Anya Hindmarch evening bag.

It's going to be soon. I can feel it in the fragrance of the moon, which is somehow earthier. It's as if the moon is carrying with it the smells of earth that are quite different from the smells up here. I can smell jasmine, which is the smell of fertility, so definitely it's going to be soon.

Falling and falling, I'm drawn to this new life with a sense of delightful abandon, like sunflowers are drawn to the sun and swallows are drawn to the warm South. After years of adult analysing, it seems we happen upon a path and the most sensible thing to do is just to meander along it. Enjoy the smell of the flowers and take special note of the cloud formations. Wherever the destination is, it's like love preordained by higher beings who must be wiser than even we consider ourselves.

In a funny way, in leaving things to chance, or fate, as it were, the freedom of that free fall gives a girl a sense of security. I've done whatever I can; now, more than anything else in the world, I want to be Tallulah Xenopoulos, beloved daughter of Jason and Rahla. It seems like just about everyone on earth is madly excited with longing for me — all I have to do is turn up.

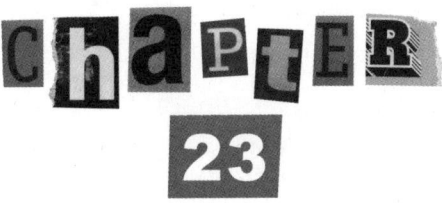

CHAPTER 23

Counting sheep

And, after patiently waiting and waiting, after an intolerable forever, I found myself tossing and turning with only one sleep to go …

12 p.m. midnight
It is utterly unbearable. For the first time in forever I wish I could pop just half a sleeping pill. Instead of giving my nerves and body a rest, my brain is running riot and going amok in a frenzy of over-activity … it won't do, it won't do. I implore the universe, God, myself, please let me sleep and dream of sheep.

2.30 a.m.
Even the dogs aren't moaning. The whole house is peacefully slumbering, joyfully ignorant of my wide-awake torment. I drink mugs

of Horlicks and cups of chamomile tea. I read the dictionary, count sheep and say at least a dozen Hail Marys. I say thank-yous to God for each and every act of kindness and good humour that has been bestowed on me for all the thirty-six years of my life. I pray to the lord God Jah, to Hashem, to Allah and to Steve Biko.

Maybe, I think, if I take just a quarter of a sleeping pill, would that be dangerous? Would Tallulah then fall asleep inside my tummy for another hundred years? Waiting there until a handsome prince could wade through all the forests and bones to kiss her awake and into a fairy-tale world? I grow afraid that the nap she is having inside me may become all too restful with even a quarter of a pill. No, no, no. I say twenty *om mani padme hums* that ought to lull me into a gentle, meditative Buddhist slumber and out of my wide-awake state of vexation.

I've always suffered from insomnia; when I was younger, I rarely slept at all. Falling asleep was a time-consuming drag, and once I was asleep it was a delicate rest, easily disturbed. My father suffered similarly, and as my head finally submitted to the pillow I'd often hear him coming up the passageway. With a twinkle in his voice, he'd say, 'I'm an insomniac but I don't lose any sleep over it.' Then he'd go upstairs to spend hours of silent intrigue in his study wall-papered with books, leaving me to lie bored and awake.

4.30 a.m.
Picking away at the morose morsels lodged deep inside the bowels of my crazy brain. By now it is too late to take a pill anyway, and I know that I ought to be grateful because this 10 000-hour-long night is coming to a point of dawn. A mere three hours and the frenetic loneliness of it all will be slaughtered by the joy and noise of dawn breaking. Just three hours to go till the Monday of blood tests and results. I remind myself over and over again that Tallulah

or no Tallulah, the orchid in the garden will flower, and that that in itself is a wondrous thing. And yet, the suspense is unbearable. '*Ommm mani padme hummmm, ommm mani padme hummmmm …* Hail O jewel in the flower of the lotus, hail.' And hail sanity, hail morning, hail evening, hail Jason, love of my little life, hail Tallulah, hail the promise of dawn and hail the sanity of a new day.

5 a.m.

Finally, dawn. The HOOhu hooROOhuhu of a dove sounding like an owl on speed. Or is it just voices making a cacophony of chaos in my brain?

CHAPTER 24

Tallulah safe and sound

It's dark in here, dark and warm, like a caramel-coated living room. A capsule of yummy gooey stuff. It's been twelve years since the night I spotted my new mother and father meet and fall in love. That's twelve years of praying and waiting and observing. I think I've earned a good rest, a sleep of meringues and cream. I think I'll sleep like this for about eight months and sixteen days. I'm going to sleep and dream of sheep.

All the tranquillity in here makes me forgetful. I don't know if it was the journey or just being here safely, but I'm forgetting things. I can't locate stuff inside my brain. Where did I put that other memory anyway? My last recall of the crystal forest — I know it's inside here somewhere, or did I leave it behind?

Faces from other lives, numbers, ideas, names I knew a moment ago;

vroom, it's all leaving me now, and I don't really care. I'm footloose and fancy-free, starting all over again. I do hope I've packed all my important characteristics. I can't remember if the boys made it along and I can't see anything because I'm all groggy, and after the rainbows and iridescent radiance of heaven, I can't make anything out in the darkness. It doesn't matter; nothing matters now. I'm here, safe as houses in my mummy's tummy, and nothing else in the entire world exists.

In ten days' time Rahla and Jason will go for a scan and they'll take a picture of me, but I'll sleep through the moment when they get their first sight of me. Fast asleep and dreaming of a new life, I am the luckiest fish in the world. Yay for me, yay for everybody!

CHAPTER 25

Hurly-burly

Waiting and waiting. I thought it would never end and the suspense was unbearable. After that awful night in purgatory, I endured a morning of dull agitation. After the blood tests, I wandered around the shops like a bored housewife. I ate a packet of dried mango but that didn't help, so I tried rice cakes, which were tasteless.

I felt dull, numb and surprisingly despondent. I rushed home and phoned the Stork Doctor – too early; the results weren't ready yet. The morning meandered along at its own tedious pace. I tried eating toast with Marmite but found it too salty, so I tried a carrot muffin, which was too sweet.

I went for a walk to the local deli, but on the way I found the view of Table Mountain and the Atlantic Ocean irritating in its perfection, so I dawdled home to phone the Stork Doctor again. Still no news. I ate five soya sausages and locked myself in my Wendy house, hiding behind the 'depressed curtains', the strands and strands of glass beads threaded together when I was too depressed to do anything else.

Then I heard Jason screaming and shouting inside the house. By way of response to the excitement I crouched down in a foetal position, hiding from any news, good or bad. The shouting found me, getting louder and turning into raucous laughter. I opened the door of the Wendy house to find Jason standing there with a face as white as Brad Pitt's teeth, and I realised he was talking to the Stork Doctor on the cellphone.

Rings on my fingers, bells on my toes, elephants to ride upon, my little Irish rose, I was pregnant!

I remember being sixteen years old, standing with my best friend in the upstairs ladies' section of the *shul*, the two of us looking down on all the *yarmulkaed* heads bopping to and fro in prayer. Naturally the boys were of far more relevance to us than religion. The *boys* were our religion. It was Erev Rosh Hashanah, the night before the beginning of the New Year.

Looking at a particularly sexy and inspiring *yarmulkaed* head, I said to my friend, 'Let's make this the best year of our lives.' Laughing, she agreed, and we continued to watch that appealing, now-forgotten boy. The funny thing is that I don't remember who the boy was or how the year transpired – just the wacky, infatuated hopefulness.

The Monday that I found out I was pregnant I thought to myself, maybe this year at Rosh Hashanah I'll lug my lazy, irreligious ass over to *shul* and thank God for it all. I can't remember if I got there or not, but it's doubtful. Oy, the promises we make.

There's so much beauty in the world. Some days it's uplifting, and other days it's almost sad in its beauty and it can drag you down, 'down down where the iguanas play'. But whatcha gonna do? It is as it should be and God is in His universe.

Time passed and Rosh Hashanah drew near. My belly grew and I kept on listening to Leonard Cohen complaining in his melancholy old way. I'd get me a new, new year, the best year yet. And, who knows, a tiny inkling of cheeky thought wondered, maybe the laughing old man, the suicidal urges and the desolate mood wouldn't come knocking. Except that I knew they would. That's the thing about my life. The seasons keep changing, the carousel keeps turning, madly turning, the tide goes out and comes in and yes, my mood soars up and it crashes down.

I don't really get science and evidently it doesn't really get me, either. Doctors had warned me of the life-threatening dangers of going off medication and conceiving a child. Doctors had told us that Jason was absolutely incapable of reproducing. I had researched surrogacy, adoption and sperm donors. I had at times felt such violently desperate maternal urges that I considered pilfering friends' children. One healthy child would have been the answer to all my prayers.

Life has expected a lot from me, and I expect a lot right back. When the doorbell rings on an average Monday morning, I automatically assume it's a stranger sending flowers. Great expectations! So it takes an awful lot to surprise me, but after all the medical setbacks, even I was impressed at my first scan when not one, but two little black blobs appeared on the screen.

Imagine my astonishment a few weeks later when I looked at the obstetrician's screen and saw a *third* sea monkey, who had been shyly hiding behind one of the others in the first scan. Three heartbeats. As certain as the science that had assured me I'd never have a child, Tallulah had brought along the whole jolly kindergarten!

Such was Jason's shock that for two weeks he couldn't articulate in anything that remotely resembled the English language. I'd say, 'Honey, would you like muesli for breakfast?' And his response would be, 'Aaaghvllupp brupbrupbrup oi fuck!'

Don't get me wrong; I was also in shock. The night after the revealing scan I lay in the bath and cried into the phone to a friend, 'But how will I feed and educate three children?' She sensibly said, 'Don't worry, children bring their own money.' Frankly, I don't know how Jason's pulled it off, but today we're all well fed, cared for and clothed.

A few days into the pregnancy, the morning sickness kicked in: morning, noon, night, midnight and 3 a.m. sickness. Each little sea monkey produced his or her own progesterone, which produced its own nausea. And so it was that for three months I hurled and hurled and hurled. Thanks be to God I'd had some practice as a bulimic.

About two weeks into the pregnancy I got the smarts and set up office in the bathroom. I sat hunched over the toilet bowl, notebook, mineral water and telephone placed neatly on the floor. Every page or so I'd lean over, hurl my guts out, wipe my mouth, take a sip of water and resume writing.

Three months into the pregnancy the vomiting stopped and I began to grow and grow and grow. I started looking like Demis Roussos in drag. I had to wear stretch caftans. A friend made special clothes for me; they were so outrageously large that I could hire them out as marquees for weddings and bar mitzvahs. The mere fact that I was vertical, let alone walking about, was in itself gravity-defying. It was a wonder I didn't topple over. Early in the pregnancy I became too large to reach the steering wheel of my car, so I stopped driving.

At the beginning of my first trimester Cape Town experienced a heat wave, so I moved office into the swimming pool. I paddled my gargantuan form about with notebook, water and telephone balanced on the skirting of the pool. As I dunked my head under water, then wrote and looked out at the awesome Atlantic Ocean, I mused over what a wonderful life it had turned out to be. It was as if, physically, my entire life had been a preparation for my pregnancy. All the years of dancing, doing yoga, weight training and walking made carrying an extra thirty-five kilos a no-strain situation. What should have been a high-risk pregnancy spent monitored in hospital and on bed rest was in fact eight of the happiest, most chilled, mango-bingeing, gentle, happy-hormone months of my life.

One day my gynaecologist said, 'You know, I always say people who experience life-threatening illnesses have easier lives.' For a second I thought, 'How trite. I wish I'd known how much easier my life was when I was having my stomach pumped.' But he was right. Previous illness had given me the perspective to appreciate my pregnancy for the magnificent gift that it was. I genuinely didn't feel any of the discomfort. I felt nothing but amusement and joy. It was a pregnancy of milk and honey. I hurled, laughed, ate, walked, wrote, danced, gardened, dreamt, loved and anticipated through eight blissful months. And in those eight months I could never have imagined, in my wildest dreams, what a magnificent treat lay in store for me.

The Friday before the babies were born I waddled on the beach collecting shells, then went home and did gym. On Saturday evening Jason came home from Saudi Arabia, where he'd been shooting for a month. On Sunday we went to see *The Motorcycle Diaries*, then had lunch and did some shopping.

At 5 a.m. on Monday 28 February, the day of the Oscars, I woke Jason and said, 'I've just made a huge wee in the bed!'

That day marked exactly thirty-four weeks of pregnancy. Gidon's waters had broken. He wasn't waiting another minute. We woke Livicky and, giggling hysterically, the three of us packed a hospital bag and charged out the front door as the alarm clock assigned to wake Jason and get him on a flight to Johannesburg beep-beeped to an empty house.

At the hospital I insisted to doctors and specialists that I wouldn't have my babies until I'd had a bikini wax, a wheat-free/sugar-free carrot cake and a mineral face spray. I insisted that my babies couldn't come into the world if classical music wasn't playing in the theatre at the time. Agitated nurses unceremoniously came at me with disposable razors and determined doctors approached with large epidural needles.

I often wonder whether Gidon yanked the other two out or whether Layla Tallulah was pushing Gidon and pulling Samuel. Possibly Samuel, in his quiet, persuasive manner, gave the other two a giant shove and sent them both, startling, into life. Mostly, I picture little Samuel dozing peacefully and being rudely awakened by Gidon's insistence that they all come out into the world prematurely. However it was that the three of them had their birth order arranged, at 8.30 a.m. they arrived in this world – Gidon Greg, then Layla Tallulah and, finally, Samuel Jacob: thirty fingers, thirty toes, six ears and three noses. Three teeny-weeny perfectly perfect human beings.

As out of control as my life has generally been, I'd been presumptuous enough to make plans, believing myself to be the puppeteer of my universe. Hah! The universe gave me some perspective in the control department. I was not the decider of sexes, numbers or dates of birth, or, most important of all, the personalities of my children. From day dot, they have reminded me of the power of surrender.

Cycles being what they are and humans being the romantics we are, I secretly made the assumption once again that I was cured. I convinced myself that pregnancy and childbirth had healed me.

And for a while, it did. It was a good few months before I even needed medication.

Dreams fail us, and dreams so grand that it never even occurs to us to dream them come true. Sometimes more than our wildest imaginings are realised, but still, certain realities endure. The rich get richer, the poor get poorer. Wedge heels go out of fashion and just when you've given yours away, they come back in. Politicians break promises and moods are seldom stable. The world goes round and round, drifting as it does through space. Cycles continue.

I get happy in the extreme, and I also get sad in the extreme. I have the gift of a great outrageous love, doting friends, good family, wonderful children and a sense of humour that carries me through. I have so much that will always carry me through.

Here I am, years later, same time of year, same music. Different home, different view; in fact, no view. Instead, I have a garden for children to play in. Livicky lives down the road and Pnina lives next door. I'm not the same person I was when I sat alone in a hotel room and first started writing about my life. Some days a familiar sadness encroaches on my enchanted universe, a parasite insidiously eating away at my life. Happiness leaks out of my being. Then I take to bed, go into hiding. The children go on outings with kind friends and relatives; Livicky and the staff step in.

No matter how much water I drink, my mouth remains parched. Tears and terror constantly reinvent themselves inside me, threatening violently to erupt. On those days the tears are so much a part of my being that they seem to have manifested in my bones. I imagine that long after my body, memories, words and dreams have disintegrated, my skeleton of bones with its tears and melancholy will remain. It seems that my legacy won't be my children or my words, but rather this torment.

Once more the sound of dogs barking petrifies me. The phone's ringing rakes through me like fingernails on a blackboard. I avoid eye contact with the cashier at the supermarket. I can't talk to anyone I love, because then I'll break down entirely. Little daily rituals and routines are monstrous, unachievable tasks.

Life overwhelms me and the sadness creates a malevolent screen between my children and me. I watch them playing in the garden. Learning to walk, babbling and gurgling at one another in a language understandable only to them, a language they must have created in the womb. They laugh and discover the brand-new world in a courtyard underneath a lemon tree. Watching, I'm ashamed of my pain.

All my dreams have come idyllically true. Is this sadness so great that it's even greater than them? Can it consume the sight of these wondrous children? But still, the tears flow. If only someone would phone with good news, if a bouquet of flowers would be delivered, if Amazon would courier a book I hadn't ordered. I'm waiting for something to happen to lift the weight of the pain. Then I remember – there is nothing that helps.

Delicately I pick and pick away at the peripheral padlock of pain, and then, poof, there it is, a blunt knife stabbing right into the heart of the matter. There's nothing, the anxiety, it doesn't come from out there, it comes from within. No matter how good the going gets, this illness will always be lurking, waiting. The monkey on my back, the thorn in my side, the pain in my neck, the black dog barking at my door. The laughing, mocking, sinister voice of the old man reminding me not to get too confident, reminding me that there's no cure for what I'm feeling.

There may be days, weeks, months even, of light and life restored to me. Times when I feel like an ordinary girl, a kind of remission in a long-term incurable illness. But always, the good times are punctuated by this cycle of despair. It never ends; it never goes away and *stays* away.

And I know this feeling all too well – I've walked this line so many times, carried myself across this dark, forlorn highway. I know every headlight and curve of the road. I know when to be aware of oncoming traffic and when to slow down for the traffic police. It all floods over me like a delayed and unhelpful moment of déjà vu. It seems I've trodden this particular journey since time immemorial. And no matter how familiar the black highway might be, it still assaults me with undiminished pain. The same old story, the same pain, but fresh as new, regenerating and regenerating the anguish.

Each night as my head hits the pillow, I promise myself that tomorrow I will bring myself to phone the necessary doctors, lie still for the needles going in to bring mood relief. Tomorrow I will swallow the pills that make me fat and scramble my brain. I will gag as I swallow, but I know how to stomach the potions.

Tomorrow I will stretch every limb of my body, force myself to exercise, charge up and down the mountainside so fast that I don't notice the view from the top. Tomorrow I will try to cut out the causes of stress in my life even if they bring me much-needed pleasure. I will say at least ten *om mani padme hum*s and bathe in essence of clary sage. I will try not to spend time alone even if I desperately need my solitude and, just in case, just in case, I will double-check all the medication in the household – because you never really know, do you?

Tomorrow, terrified and alone, I will leave my children, get on a plane and fly to Johannesburg to see the Happy Potter doctor. If needs be, I will be checked into hospital and I will sleep alone in a ward among the crazy and despairing until my medications are tweaked, the danger passes, my mood shifts and I'm fit to live in the world again.

It may get better, it may very well get worse, but eventually, as my mother always says, 'It will pass.'

Epilogue

I raise my head from the page, turning to look out into the garden through the open half of the stable door, and there, in the dappled shade of the lemon tree, is my husband with our three treasures. The truffles. Our triplets. My little tribe.

I imagine that maybe Tallulah couldn't decide whom she wanted to play with the most, so she brought both beloved brothers along. Of course, being children and not remote-controlled fantasies, they came with their own distinct and perfect personalities.

Sometimes when my little girl gazes at us with her penetrating, curious stare, raising her right eyebrow in amusement, my mother goes quite cold, because it is my father's gaze. Other days, I watch Tallulah clanking down the road wearing a green velvet ball gown, pink hat and Pnina's green Manolo Blahnik stilettos. Then I think, dear God, I've given birth to my sister, all glamorous and stylish.

And sometimes, when Gidon Greg, my big boy, shrieks with excitement, wriggles with joy, laughs for no apparent reason, gets lost in a reverie listening to Pachelbel's *Canon* while studying dinosaur books, when he invites me into the fantasy world where he spends so much time, a world inhabited by dragons and fantasy 'brothers', he reminds me of the glorious magnificence of his late uncle's craziness, the much-missed, much-loved Greg.

The littlest baby, Samuel Jacob, the last one to come out of my tummy, is dark and brooding. Quite an eccentric little magnet, he seems to provoke adoration from the most unlikely sources. His hair is coiled into black spirals like the night sky in Van Gogh's *Starry Night*. He has a wicked sense of humour, and his black eyes have the same gentle allure as his father's.

I've come to think that we reincarnate in the lives of our children. We, or aspects of each of us, are carried through time on this earth in our children and our children's children. Mind you, they are who they are today, but they may change completely by next week. However, I doubt that they will ever be anything other than perfect.

What delights and astonishes me is that we don't merely live to tell the tale. We live to watch movies, gossip with girlfriends, spend mornings gardening and afternoons gazing out at the ocean as white sails cruise languidly by. We live to love and laugh and cry and reproduce and read and write and make love and eat popcorn and drink green tea and sit as families around Georgian dining-room tables. To light candles and thank whatever gods may be out there for our unconquerable souls, and to bask in the great glow of faith.

Glossary

bene	good
bashert	fate
Erev Rosh Hashanah	the night before Jewish New Year
kibbutz	communal, collective agricultural settlement in Israel
kibbutzniks	people living on a kibbutz
manyana	tomorrow
mensch	good human being
om mani padme hum	Buddhist mantra seeking enlightened awareness
Oise Yom Tov	the good days are over

petlach	bags
Rosh Hashanah	Jewish New Year
safta	grandmother
schlep	drag, to lug something with difficulty
schmutsik	dirty
Shabbat	Sabbath
Shen Men	gateway for the spirit
shiva	period of mourning
shul	synagogue, place of worship
tokoloshe	hairy phantom being of African folklore
tschatskes	little ornaments, toys, playthings
verlep	withered
vershtunkende	stinking
yarmulka	Jewish skullcap